posture power
for women

Carol has taken an innovative approach in bringing this subject back into focus. She is being very creative in developing a unique practice, with posture and wellness integrated, with the end result being a happy patient who has had a fun experience with lasting results in a changed lifestyle.

Peter A. Towne, PT, Chair, International Private Practitioners
Association of Physical Therapists, USA

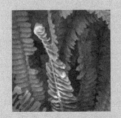

posture power
for women

Carol Armitage

with Mike Bebb

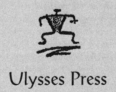

Ulysses Press

Published by Ulysses Press
       P.O. Box 3440
       Berkeley, CA 94703
       www.ulyssespress.com

ISBN: 1-56975-475-6
Library of Congress Catalog Number: 2005922411

First published as *The Power of Posture* in New Zealand in 2003
   by Random House New Zealand

Printed in Canada

10 9 8 7 6 5 4 3 2 1

Interior design and layout: Christine Hansen
Cover design: Leslie Henriques
Cover photograph: © Jupiterimages.com
U.S. editorial and production: Lynette Ubois, Steven Schwartz,
   Nicholas Denton-Brown, Lily Chou
Indexer: Sayre Van Young
Photographs: Bernadette Peters
Author photograph on page 144: Graeme Brown
Illustrations: Anne Heng
Digital images (section heads and chapter openers): Kathy Glentworth

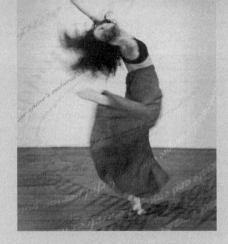

CONTENTS

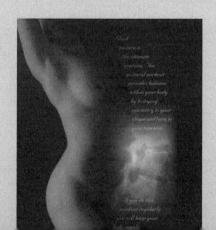

SECTION THREE: POSTURE IS PERSONAL

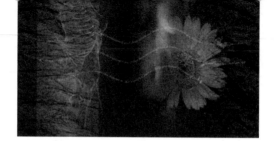

ACKNOWLEDGEMENTS

What a journey this book has taken me on – which somehow, I feel is just beginning. I am indebted to many wonderful people in my life, some of whom are mentioned here.

Special thanks to Dr. Mike Bebb, Ph.D., who encouraged me to create my own vision: you showed me how to live my life with purpose and paint my own canvas. To the incredibly talented photographer Bernadette Peters, the fantastically creative graphic designer Kathy Glentworth, and the illustrator of the exquisite drawings Anne Heng, who together breathed life and soul into the manuscript with the stunning images – what a team.

I thank the team at Random House, especially Christine Thomson, who simply is the best in the business, and editors Pat Field and Kim O'Keefe, and designer Christine Hansen. To Steve Barnett: thank you, you believed in the book right from the start.

Thanks to all the fabulous women, children and dogs who delighted us with their portrayal of the true power of posture, and to all the cafés and businesses around my city of Palmerston North, New Zealand, who allowed us to shoot the pictures around them as they were working. Especially Ihi Aotearoa, Studio Astoria, Barista's, and Cook Street Nursing Home.

The artwork on page 112 is by Denise Tohiariki (Ngati Raukawa).

And thanks heaps to my colleagues through the years who have become such great friends. Sarah Dewes: thanks for the weekend when we brainstormed women's health issues and other topics. To Anne Williams, who kept my clinic going through the last few years of this book, along with my work mates, and to Dr. O'Leary for his undoubting support (Yes, I actually did it!).

And to my clients who, every day, provide me with much joy and laughter.

To the heroes of my life: thank you for your inspiration.

And I acknowledge my biggest fans, Paul, Zachary, Jessica and Arielle, it is really the other way around guys – I love you.

Carol

My first awareness of the real power of posture was in performing gymnastics, especially stepping out across the mat and taking up the pose that began my routine (today, my body still has a perfect memory of that position). The judges, the audience, my coach and parents would be totally focused on me. It was not like having to jump the highest or run the fastest, but more conveying a certain quality of movement. I would try to set the scene, control the atmosphere and project my personality all before the music began – even if I was trembling inside.

I had exciting mentors in gymnastics. I have trained with Olympic champions, and I know the thrill of competing for your country. There were hours and hours spent trying to emulate these great athletes and I know now that this training in my formative years shaped my attitude to the sheer presence and power of posture.

My professional training and life's work as a physiotherapist has taught me the significance of posture and the clinical reasoning behind the effects it has on our bodies and minds. It helped me to place posture in a medical context and develop a fascination for anatomy and the mechanics of movement. I already knew how training affected movement and the patterns we call habits, but I also began to understand the effects of self-esteem and emotions.

For over 20 years I have worked in the area of sports rehabilitation. This has given me considerable opportunities to understand the wear and tear from competitive sport, and the intensity that is required to prepare for international competition. My work with elite athletes in many sports taught me the value of learning self-awareness through body alignment and posture.

I became interested in creating self-awareness and decreasing the effects of stress for everyone, particularly in my specialty area of women's health. Most people seldom think about posture and many freely admit they have bad posture (that's why they send their daughters to ballet, they tell me). And I was beginning to learn how to express and see myself more deeply, not as a gymnast, physiotherapist, but as a whole person – me.

As a mother of three children I have felt some of the changes women's bodies experience through pregnancy, birth and the demanding years when children are small ... I hope this book will empower all women to use good posture to make their lives more stress-free, joyous and fulfilling.

INTRODUCTION

Across a crowded room, suddenly you become aware of a person that you not only see, but feel and almost taste – and instantly you are aware of how alive you are … The way people communicate their very being is a powerful message. Stating who we are, what we want and even what we stand for actually happens without saying a word. An intuitive form of socialization is people-watching. We all take part in it, whether we are aware of it or not. If people were watching you right now, what would you be saying to them with your body language or postural language?

Your posture is your physical signature. It portrays your uniqueness and is a very personal script used to communicate with others. With posture you can project yourself, reflect your attitudes and enhance your self-esteem, making a far deeper and longer-lasting impression than the shiniest hair or the whitest smile. Your posture is really stature. Great stature means having positive self-awareness, not just a toned body. The power of posture in essence is expressing your personality physically.

Good posture is very energizing and clearly has enormous benefits for the health of your body: it protects you while you move and when you are stationary because it aligns your spine and joints; it creates balance in the way your muscles work and gives symmetry to your shape; it helps support internal organs and enhances sexual responsiveness; and it uses your energy stores more efficiently. As your posture improves and good habits replace sloppy ones, this will impact on such things as back pain, headaches or slack tummy muscles and lead to a greater sense of well-being.

For a lot of women today good posture seems unrealistic. Our lifestyles are making us slouch over computers and sit for long periods of time and even our children are exercising less. But it doesn't take a lifetime of vigorous training and drills to develop good posture – it just requires a subtle balance within your body. This balance will enable you to move with grace and beauty, to remain active through your life and enjoy a healthy and happy body.

While improving your posture may be your present goal, I wish it to last longer than after you have walked past the first full-length mirror. Becoming in tune with your body through your posture will help you to feel the youthfulness of life for your entire life. As well as a physical "ironing out of the creases," postural improvement will enhance the emotional and spiritual feelings you have about yourself. Just like your smile, your posture will radiate the inner you.

My life's work and passion as a physiotherapist is to help you to achieve all this. I invite you to use the principles in this book to create a body you can be really proud of. Perhaps your biggest challenge is to believe that you are worth it, to find your strength in the power of posture. This book will give you the opportunity to:

- learn about and realize for yourself the benefits of good posture.
- gain a vision of the woman you would like to be.
- give yourself a simple body assessment, so you can see where you are physically in relation to your goals.
- begin to attain your vision by using good posture as your secret weapon.
- get into the posture workout – an exercise script to keep all parts of your body in fine working order over your lifetime.
- add in special extra exercises designed to combat the changes brought about by age, illness and injury.

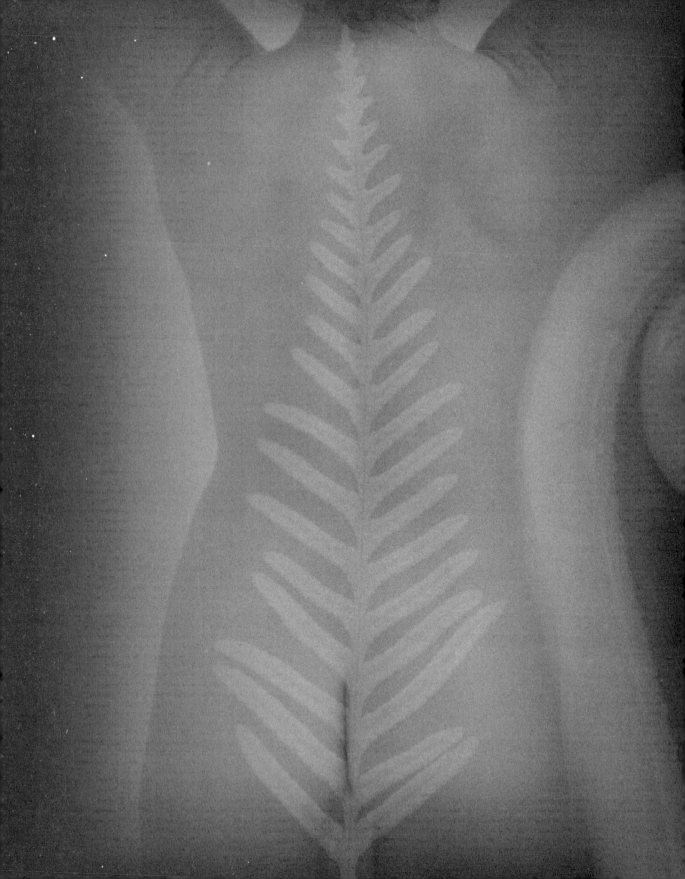

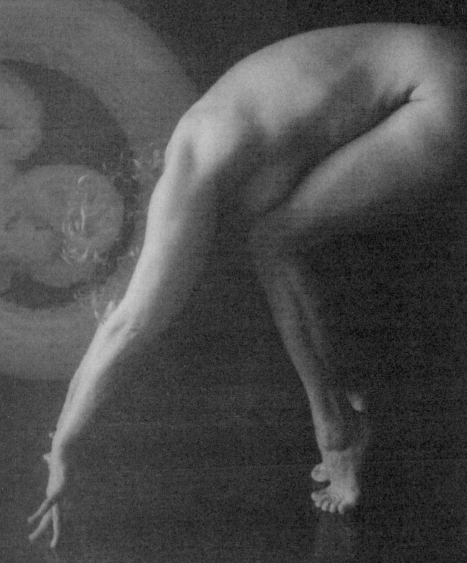

The way people communicate their very being is a powerful message. Stating who we are, what we want and even what we stand for actually happens without saying a word.

Your posture is your physical signature. It portrays your uniqueness and is a very personal script we use to communicate with others. With posture you can project yourself, reflect your attitudes and enhance your self-esteem, making a far deeper and longer lasting impression than the shiniest hair or the whitest smile. Your posture is really stature. Great stature means having a positive self awareness, its not just a toned body. The power of posture in essence is expressing your personality physically.

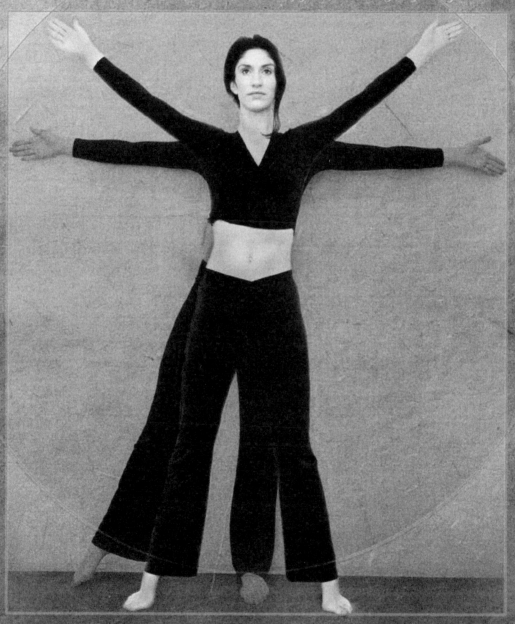

The lower torso section (tummy) and pelvic floor platform (underneath and deep inside us) make up the unique part of a woman. Not only does this part of us hold the key - in a postural sense - to our bodies, but also throughout time it has been associated with a women's physical, emotional and even spiritual energy. Influencing and directing the changes that happen to this essential part will help you to feel the power of posture.

Chapter 1

WHAT IS GOOD POSTURE?

The lower torso section (tummy) and pelvic floor platform (underneath and deep inside us) make up the unique part of a woman. Not only does this part hold the key – in a postural sense – to our bodies, but also throughout time it has been associated with a woman's physical, emotional and even spiritual energy. Influencing and directing the changes that happen to this essential part will help you to feel the power of posture.

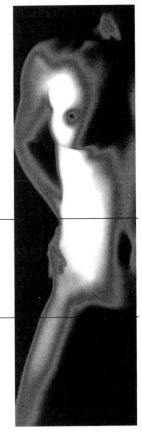

Many women despair at the look, feel and shape of themselves through this midsection, especially after childbirth or as they hit 40! Beautiful posture will define and tone this part of your body to enhance your natural sensuousness as a woman.

Initially you may think improving your posture is about sticking your shoulders back and thrusting your breasts forward. This is not so. Great posture comes by continually lifting up from this lower torso region, creating a balance and grace in your body that can be very empowering – see what I mean by trying these simple enhancements of your body position:

Whatever your position right now, sitting, lying or standing, place your fingers on your hip bones and thumbs on your lower ribs. Then elongate the space in between, lift and lengthen your abdominal wall, like stretching a concertina. Don't hunch your shoulders or hold your breath, don't even move your shoulders or chest, just try to lift up and out of your inner center ... Doesn't that feel powerful?

When you are next walking, try to repeat this awareness exercise to "own the feeling." Feel where this energy comes from. Don't think about anything important or unpleasant. Float along, drawing up and out from the core of your being, this area between your belly button and pelvis. You will feel you could walk for hours.

Keeping your head level and your eyes looking forward, lengthen the space between your collarbones and chin.

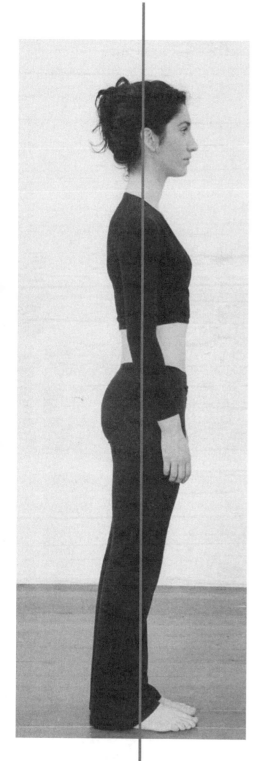

*Feel the space between your chin and chest. Make sure
you relax your body so that you can hold it effortlessly.*

Improving your posture with these two simple actions anytime, anywhere will develop a strong support for your body.

You may know you have poor posture, but just what is good posture? Most of us had perfect posture as a child, then life experiences and influences such as injuries, illnesses, genetic inheritances, aging and work habits alter and erode the perfect shape, sculpting us into individuals. Your unique characteristics make you special. Good posture is not about bringing back the perfect form, but developing a strong energy and power base.

If you observe people with no postural awareness, you can almost see a heavy chain around their necks pulling them down and forward, as if they were carrying the weight of the world on their shoulders. A feeling of having too big or too small breasts, being too tall or lacking confidence can make women sink down into their chests and become round shouldered, which can lead to chronic pain in the upper back. Further down the body, faulty posture from poor abdominal and pelvic floor muscle tone can result in stiff joints in the spine, hips or legs.

*While standing (when you are feeling fresh, not when you are
tired and starting to sag), feel the hollow in the small of your
back, and a similar one just behind your neck. The idea is to keep
these curves when you stand, walk, or sit.*

A SIDE VIEW OF GOOD POSTURE

Classic good posture in women is not about straight lines, but supporting your spine's natural curves. Don't worry about a sway back or a flat back unless you have difficulty moving freely or are in discomfort or pain.

To get an idea of ideal posture, viewed from the side, imagine a marker on your ears, the ends of your shoulders and the middle of the side of your hips; a plumb line dropped from vertical should fall through these points. When standing, the plumb line would also fall through markers placed on the outside of your knees and ankles.

Whatever you are doing, keep these points of reference in the back of your mind. Sitting and leaning forward, walking or running should be done with the first three imaginary markers all in line. Keeping these key parts of your body in one line, with your body curving around it, will place your neck and shoulders in a neutral position. This doesn't take any extra time but does save you energy by protecting your spine and using your muscles correctly. Sagging this plumb line will place undue stress on your body.

POSTURE IN ACTION

The human body in action follows a complex pattern of activity involving the brain, spine, muscles and joints. Well-trained athletes have incredible postural control centering from their torso. Holding the trunk firm is a very efficient way to generate speed, leap high or hold exquisite balance. Holding your body firm as you go through your day will allow you to achieve a similar efficiency in your movement.

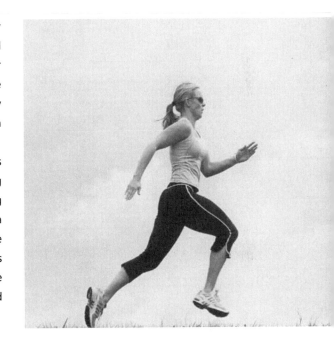

As an example, bending is a movement we all do hundreds of times a week. Bending with good posture involves tipping forward from the hips, placing your buttocks out and bending from the knees. This places your body in an optimal position for lifting, using your thighs, even in an awkward position like getting kids in and out of car seats. Bending from your hips with your torso held firm and keeping those markers in line will help prevent problems such as backache, sore neck and headaches and you will not tire so easily.

AVOID BAD HABITS

You may work in a situation that requires you to lean over or bend forward, such as nursing, or sit at a desk looking at a computer screen all day or, like most mothers, work physically hard carrying, lifting and stooping. Just being tired all the time can cause you to sag emotionally as well as physically. If you are in pain or in distress you tend to curl down and around yourself, and while this may be temporary it can also become a long-term habit. In a very short time the tendency, especially when you are busy, is to not straighten up fully and keep those plumb lines correct. Over time it becomes harder to feel or even know where the naturally correct alignment of your body is.

By becoming aware of your posture and having a positive attitude to yourself, you will not only feel, but look better. If you aim for a variety of movement in your day, include a balance of exercise and relaxation, give yourself the respect you deserve – the benefits will delight and surprise you.

BENEFITS THAT WILL REALLY LAST

Good posture accumulates many long-term benefits. I know you will want them all, but to make this relevant for you, I want you to select from the following list the three that are most personally appropriate … right this minute take a pen and check off the three that you relate to most.

- More energy
- Define who you are
- Enhance your sexuality
- Develop physical power (over your shape, your aches and pains)
- Positive aging – get older and better!

MORE ENERGY

We can all benefit from a gentle, supple, more graceful way of going about our day. The power of posture uses the natural rhythms of movement, tension and relaxation to create balance within your body, giving the effect of moving fluidly. For your body to work efficiently and so it can feel and look good, you require a blend of both muscular control and relaxation.

You can conserve energy and actually reduce the stress on your body, i.e. your ligaments and joints, by increasing the efficiency of how you go about your day. This does not mean you have to do hard workouts; by simply aligning yourself in good postural positions you will feel a lot better and create the effect of looking fabulous.

DEFINE WHO YOU ARE

Your posture is a powerful but gentle way to achieve, express, envision and create YOU. Does making a personal statement as you sit, stand and walk seem a novel idea? This benefit will become apparent to you in the form of more strength, more suppleness and more shape and control of the "not so easy to exercise" parts, like your lower tummy. When you contract a muscle it shortens, so bracing your abdominal muscles will pull your tummy in tighter, thus firming and shaping. Applied all over, and over time, you will alter your shape.

Define rather than deny yourself through dieting and excessive exercise regimes. Take a non-emotional look at yourself in the mirror and find the good parts, even some great parts of you that others love. Sometimes we just get too caught up in the body shape issue, the fat versus fabulous complex, but good posture will always outshine a not-so-perfect body size.

ENHANCE YOUR SEXUALITY

Women's sexuality is no longer just packaged and marketed to sell magazines, or hidden from most of us in books on sex therapy, or the subject of embarrassed questions to doctors. Your sexual expression is for you to explore, claim and enjoy.

Improving pelvic floor muscle tone through doing simple exercises is an intimate and personal emphasis of the power of posture, giving you the opportunity to discover facets of your femininity through physical and emotional interplay, as well as creating important life habits of bladder control and support of internal organs.

DEVELOP PHYSICAL POWER (OVER YOUR SHAPE AND YOUR ACHES AND PAINS)

Bad positional habits, such as holding a baby on one hip or standing on one leg jutting your hip out, will create poor muscle tone and shape, whereas good posture reduces many stresses that may contribute to major problems such as low back pain, head and neck aches. Ask yourself: Do you feel tired at the end of the day? Do you feel achy and stiff from what you have been doing all day? Postural control will help to prevent damage to our bodies in stressful times. The control of our body in a postural sense helps to protect it from harm, from the abuse we often put it through, such as sitting at a desk all day! You can choose to become aware of your postural habits and make them good ones.

POSITIVE AGING — GAINING CONTROL OF AGE-RELATED CHANGES

Don't underestimate the attractiveness of an older woman. As you get older you have many stories to tell – tell them with your eyes, your body language; live them through your posture, your activity, your life. You have many years to live, so live them well.

We face challenges as we feel the changes to our bodies that age brings. What can you do to improve your chances? With your body awareness through postural power, you can manage the symptoms that have a negative influence, such as bone loss, wear and tear, changes due to hormonal fluctuations, menopause and age-related changes.

There may be some issues to work through with your health professional, such as pain, but many of these are influenced by our emotional responses, triggered by our feelings. Don't let pain overwhelm you so that you stop activity and lose fitness and health. If you have pain that gets no worse with your activity, take a break, but keep going. If it gets worse or remains worse with activity, get it checked out. And remember, menopause is not forever!

Choosing the benefits you felt applied to you right now will have helped to focus your inner strength more effectively. Now I would like you to sit back comfortably and very well supported – this means your neck and spinal curves are supported and maintained without strain. Your feet should be flat on the ground, or you could elevate your legs and keep your feet free to wiggle. Feel the tension slide out of your body and the warmth that comes with this. Take a quiet moment for yourself and consider how you can claim all the benefits described above, and allow your posture to work its magic.

The following chapters will teach you all you need to know.

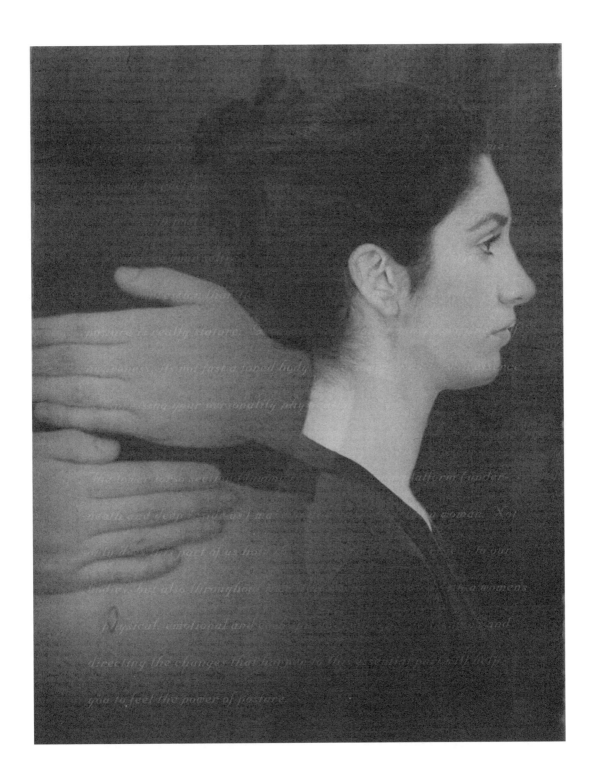

21

WHAT IS GOOD
POSTURE?

Your posture is the signature that the world sees as an expression of your personality.

Chapter 2

GET READY TO CHANGE YOUR LIFE

INTELLIGENT EXERCISE

Your first thought may be that if you did more exercise you would achieve all the benefits that the power of posture brings. While I wish you to consider the general health benefits of exercise, I would also like to make sure you choose the best strategies for you.

Back when women were not encouraged to work or do any physical exercise, and were being tied into shape with corsets, training in deportment and posture was considered a necessity. It probably was the only way a woman could be toned and keep her body relatively free of pain.

Many of us will remember being nagged by parents to "sit up straight, push your chest out, pull your shoulders back." That is probably why we all rebelled and slouching became fashionably chic.

As women become more assertive and more active, deportment and postural training is virtually non-existent. Although women today are fitter and stronger, most are working, raising children and participating in all aspects of life. This has given them a dilemma because, although they are so busy, their postures are often stationary (as in sitting over a desk) or in a fixed position (like driving). All the modern conveniences mean they do household tasks with minimum effort (unlike the way their grandmothers did), so their lifestyle has become a postural nightmare.

In my clinic I often see people with poor posture who have started exercising and ended up with back pain. And working longer hours is leading to more and more of the population suffering from tension headaches and RSI (repetitive stress injuries).

Good postural habits

Do your main daily activity keeping your plumb line upright and body held firm from your torso.

Make it a habit that you return yourself to neutral alignment. If you have to bend forward, always straighten all the way back upright.

Think active positions rather than passive positions. This means hold yourself with your muscles rather than sag onto your joints. Don't slouch, sag, or rest in sloppy positions.

Macromove. *Don't just stay in one position. When you feel yourself start to slouch or sag, get up, move around, stretch, then resume the position.*

Micromove. *Say hello to all your body parts, with a wiggle, a stretch and a squeeze to nourish them with a circulation boost. Remove waste products and pump fresh oxygen into muscles by relaxing them, moving them and releasing them from their current state of tension, e.g. rolling your shoulders, pumping ankles up and down, taking a deep belly breath. See the list on page 111 for more ways to micromove.*

Utilize breathing correctly, with belly breathing (see page 53) to help you have good oxygenation of your muscles and keep you alert but relaxed (athletes would call this focus).

DEFINING ME

Do you remember practicing your signature over and over when you were younger? The first ones had well-formed letters connected to make a beautifully written name; then over time your signature matured into this illegible scribble that you do today so that you are the only one who can reproduce it repeatedly. But isn't it you – that scribble? So too is your postural signature that the world sees as an expression of your personality.

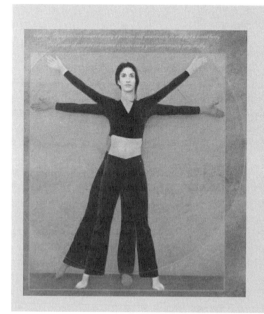

THE FOUR Ps

To define yourself as a woman and one who is in control of her body, I have developed the four Ps or principles of posture.

PORTRAY – portray a positive image of yourself which will reflect in your lifestyle.

PRACTICE – as you practice good habits of posture, this will carry over and unconsciously reflect in how you move through your day.

PROTECT – the key to protecting your body from aches and pains is good posture.

PREVENT – good posture provides you with a prevention strategy against wear and tear, for the long-term health of your body.

I am watching my daughter's cat as I write this. She embodies a sensual, controlled elegance and casual nonchalance. Cats are combinations of graceful power, slothfulness and total relaxation. This one stretches from nose to tail every time she gets up, and when she needs to jump – wow, can she jump! Good posture is a similar combination of balance within your body and is a great feeling.

Your posture is one of the most personal tools you have to create and define who you are, maybe along with your smile; the power of posture has the effect of spreading much joy. Work *with* your posture, not on your posture, to enjoy your body to its best advantage. Use your posture to send out signals to portray yourself. Like any training, good posture requires practice to create good habits, but once these are ingrained into your circuitry they will protect and prevent your body from suffering the effects of injury, illness and age-related problems.

People usually have their bodies idling in neutral, just ticking along, like a car waiting at a light. Look at everyone else as you wait in line at the supermarket checkout. What is the posture of the average man or woman? How is their body alignment, is it supportive and balanced? Do they really look as if they have their stature under control? What is their signature?

Portray

Your posture is your personal physical signature. Do not be embarrassed or lack the confidence to speak with your body; it all depends on what you want to say and after all it is the universal language. Have some fun with your posture. The whole mood of waiting in line at a supermarket can be altered by the way you stand and hand over the groceries. Simple situations can be made into classic events when you use your posture effectively.

People who love you never forget the statement you make with your body. How do your children see you and what is it about you that you wish them to respond to? As people get older, sometimes their postural signature alters as it reflects changes in their body – this is life, and can be seen as a positive change. Although we may never know exactly who we are or what we want, as we go through stages such as new motherhood, the challenge of cancer, menopause, separation, or love, the inner strength gained with self-awareness gives us the capacity to roll with the punches, and deal with the big issues of life. We can acknowledge the wisdom and beauty reflected in the changing signature in all our dimensions, physical, social, emotional and spiritual.

Practice

As you go through life, make the postural habits you develop as good as you can. Good postural habits are a conscious decision. Habits by definition become subconscious so that if you practice anything often enough you will do it without having to think about it. Then, without realizing it, you will be portraying a woman who knows who she is.

Your body, muscles, joints, spine and nervous system need to be protected from harm, fatigue, stress and injury.

To protect yourself in a postural sense, you need to consider whether you do any repetitive tasks, or tasks that place your body and health under strain. Prolonged keyboard work, sitting or standing are all risks for fatigue, stress and strain on your body. Perhaps you have to do lifting in your day. Is there a chance for you to take a break and reverse the positions that you do so often?

Work environments that make you tired and unhappy will place you at risk if you are not careful about postural fitness.

PREVENT

Future physical problems and deterioration can to a large extent be prevented. Most of the aches and pains we create in our bodies come simply from holding stationary positions for long periods of our day, or from being in similar positions repeatedly, which fatigues certain parts of us. This means there is the potential for the working body parts to shorten and get tight in some areas and lengthen and get weak in others, which can set up problems that can cause pain.

Habits of posture are often formed as adolescents develop – when their self-esteem roller coasters and body changes take effect. But think about how much bending a young mother at home with preschool children would do over a day and night. The amount of time a woman spends in the similar positions of stooping, bending and lifting throughout the day is substantial. If you are in this situation, many things can help prevent your posture becoming a problem.

BAD HABIT	GOOD HABIT
Talking on the cell phone while doing another task	Just talk on the cell phone, with your head straight
Doing your bills in bed	Bed is for relaxation
Always lying on one side of your body	Vary your positions of rest
Crossing your legs	Vary how you sit, cross your ankles
Tipping your head to one side	Check how your head rests
Carrying a bag across one shoulder	Use a backpack or two bags
Never warming up before exercise	Use a 10-minute activity as a warm-up before exercise
Standing on one leg, jutting out one hip	Stand well and evenly
Never use the back support of a chair	Always use a lumbar support
Peering closely at the computer screen	Get your vision checked
Lifting lazily, or badly	Use your legs and butt to lift

Preventing postural problems

Reverse the effects of bending too much by straightening up and extending back.

Lie or sit on the floor to read or watch TV.

Exercise your abdominals and pelvic floor muscles correctly (see exercises 2, 3, 21 and 23 in the postural workout on pages 75, 76, 96 and 97).

Always lift safely and keep your legs and low back strong (see page 49).

Keep your body fit with 30 minutes of activity a day.

Do not get too tired and remember to enjoy each day for the simplicity, chaos and joy that life surprises you with.

These four principles are important to define and to create a personal image. To clarify and focus your physical signature you must, however, do two things: 1) get rid of any excess or negative baggage; and 2) learn to trust your intuitive ability to see in pictures.

Throw away excess baggage

Gauging and examining yourself is often an emotional and negative exercise: "I hate my not-so-perfect skin, my nose is too big, I have a saggy butt … my job is not important … I'm not sexually complete …." No one is perfect. Aim to enjoy the good parts and develop the areas of yourself that don't work so well so you can reach your full potential, but please, don't go for perfection.

It's a challenge to live to your full potential. We unthinkingly limit ourselves by not getting enough activity in a balanced way so we stoop, get rounded and bent, are maybe too overweight or underweight for our health, too stiff and immobile so we get sore and grumpy, or we make ourselves wired up like a tightly coiled spring.

Do you find reasons not to do things you would like to because of lack of support, motivation or energy? Fulfilling your potential comes more easily when you create a deep and powerful vision or picture. This will provide you with courage and resilience to achieve extraordinary things.

The vision of me

"I see myself being …" Do you see words or pictures? Visions help clarify what we want and provide energy to get there. You need to let your imagination go. Visions are positive pictures – so don't fill them with getting rid of excess weight or getting rid of your sore back; rather, focus on the positive. Imagine yourself flexible, strong and fit, what you will feel, do and say when you have achieved your vision. Be bold. This is you. You are unique.

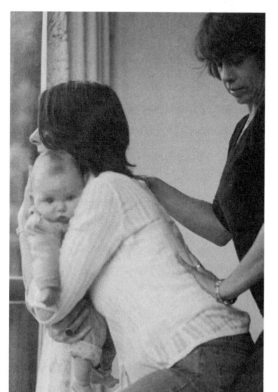

Sally's vision

Sally was a mother whose children were at school and she hated how her body, particularly her tummy, looked. She wanted to get her body more fit and desperately wanted to get back in shape. Her body had become an alien creature! Sally was in the process of writing a paper on organic gardening when she decided to identify the three improvements she hoped to see in her life (see page 18); she was initially very shy, thinking "this is silly" (just as you may be thinking now). Sally's choices were:

More energy / define who I am / enhance my sexuality.

It took courage to put down on paper her vision of herself. Sally felt embarrassed especially since she felt she couldn't draw, so she chose images instead. Her story made her vision richer, stronger and more tangible. See how simple, suggestive images and words help to develop self-confidence.

DEFINING WHO I AM

I am giving a talk to our garden group. I have successfully completed a paper on organic gardening and feel confident and passionate in sharing with my group. They enjoy the interaction as much as I do and the energy we share is huge.

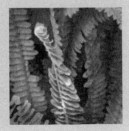

MORE ENERGY

I see myself with a smile on my face, and a spring in my step. I've walked the kids to school, I feel fit and love the feeling of boundless energy, and glances of envy. I am really alive and loving it.

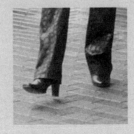

INCREASED SEXUALITY

On my phone is a message: "I've gotten a babysitter, the table is booked for 8 p.m., and we have reservations for the night at a new luxury hotel, so dress for both. I am taking you out to celebrate the sensual, wonderful woman I married 12 years ago, who I am still crazy about."

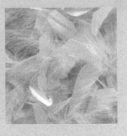

What is your ultimate story and vision for yourself? What would really light you up? Consider the three benefits you chose (see page 18) and create a masterpiece!

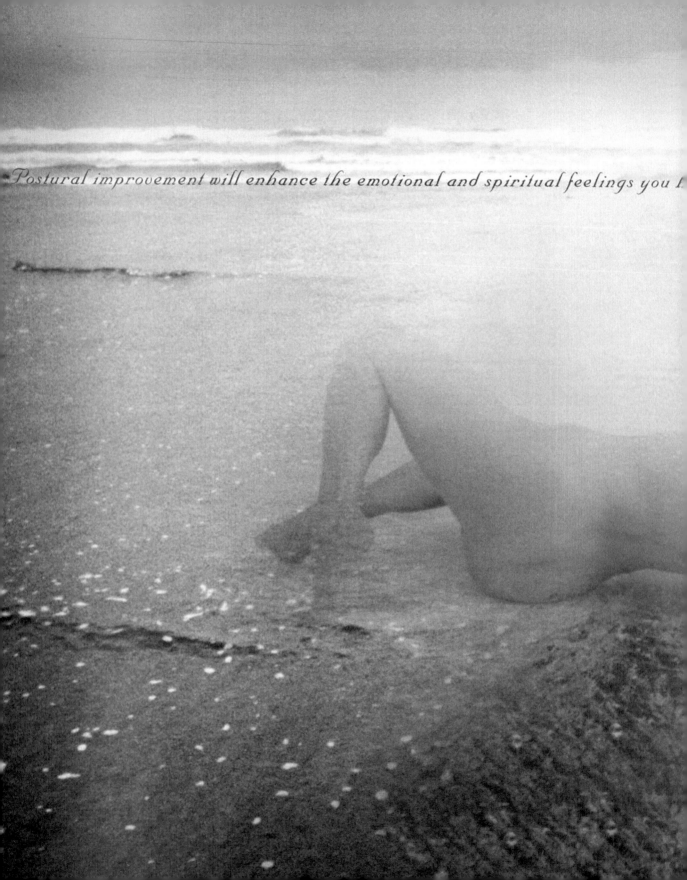

Postural improvement will enhance the emotional and spiritual feelings you h

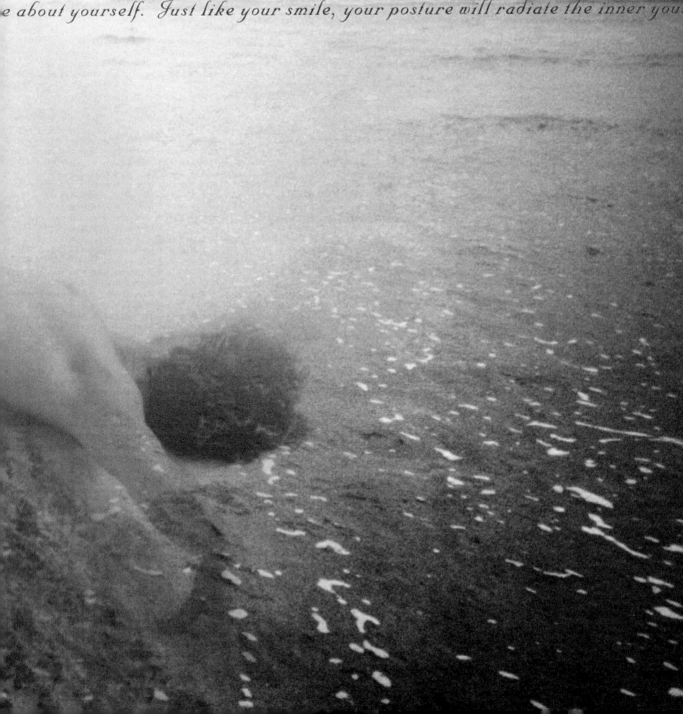

e about yourself. Just like your smile, your posture will radiate the inner you.

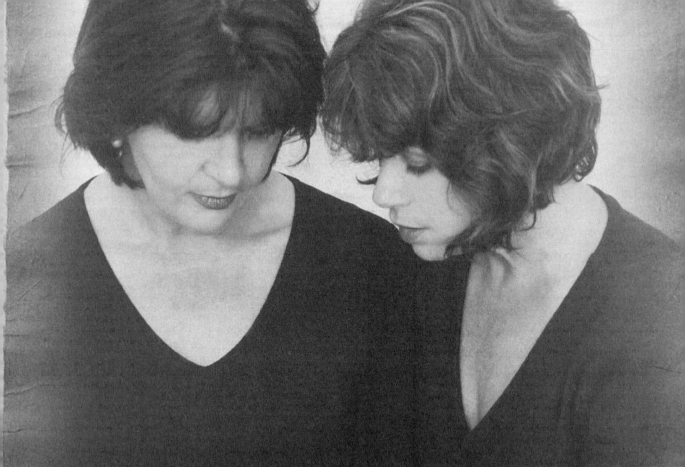

Once you can see how your posture becomes your stature, you have a very powerful tool to use. But before beginning to make any changes you need some measurements and tests.

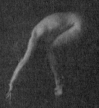
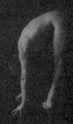
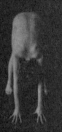

Chapter 3

ASSESSING YOUR BASIC POSTURE, FITNESS LEVEL
AND VARIETY OF ACTIVITY

Once you can see how your posture becomes your stature, you have a very powerful tool to use. But before beginning to make any changes you need some measurements and tests. You may feel your posture is good and value the ability you have to keep in shape, or you may know you need to work on your body, but are not sure where to start. Let's find out more about where you are right now. I have designed the following simple self-checks for you to do on your body:

- Basic posture in standing
- Muscle tone for women (tummy and pelvic floor muscles)
- Fitness level and variety of activity

Read through the three assessments now, try what you can, and make sure you come back to complete them before you adopt your personalized posture program.

BASIC STANDING POSTURE

One can tell a lot about a person's body and how it is working for them, simply from the way they stand. So what is your habitual posture? Is it naturally flexible and beautiful like a child's? Just how good is your basic posture in standing? This test determines whether the effects of your work and daily activities are influencing where you place your body.

> *Stand with your heels, butt and shoulder blades against a wall, facing outwards, hands by your sides. Stand in a relaxed, end-of-the-day pose.*

> *Where does your head rest? Is it against the wall or not? If not, how far does it come off of the wall, how many finger-spaces can you fit in behind your head?*

Think about this position and focus on your chest. As you stand, relax and breathe out, where is tension going out of your body – through the chest or shoulders as they sag, perhaps?

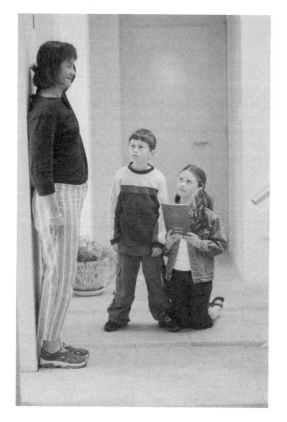

Most often the postural slump that happens with standing actually begins from your tummy being relaxed and collapsing from your chest down, like a concertina losing all its air, pulling your shoulders forward and slouching your chin forward. Ideally, I would like you to be able to rest your head easily and naturally against the back of the wall, without having to move your head back to do it, but in a lot of people the head is more like a few finger-spaces or even one fist-space away from the wall.

Children find this test easy as they naturally move in and out of postures that are not so ideal while they play and run around. As adults, we are not able to do this so readily.

Standing exercise

Lift out of your chest; don't push your breasts out, but think rather, to lift them up.

Let your shoulders fall back and down in a relaxed manner, and try to tuck your chin without tilting your head.

Slightly flatten your spine into the wall, don't bend your knees or go too far in, just feel your tummy muscles pull you toward the wall.

Try to imagine lengthening your tummy between your bottom rib and hip bones.

Reflect your vision.

You need to get the feeling of this ideal standing position. Try to take that feeling with you after you have moved away from the wall. This postural sensation is one you can adopt in any situation. It means you have the correct feeling of how to align yourself.

As you feel this, practice it often in your day, such as when you are getting ready in the morning. You can even see how you are doing by looking in the mirror.

If you find this posture difficult to sustain for longer than a few minutes, or indeed cannot feel the correct posture, you will benefit from doing exercises 8–11 of the posture workout, pages 81–89, to correct your alignment, balance and symmetry. It could be that your chest muscles have become short and tight, pulling the shoulders forward of the plumb line in relation to the back muscles which then become weak, not correctly supporting you.

MUSCLE TONE

I have taken the two vital muscle groups for women as a sample assessment for the tone of your whole body. Support and control for your posture centers from both the abdominal muscles and your pelvic floor muscles.

- Are you aware of how your tummy (abdominal) muscles need to work for you, not against you?
- Do your pelvic floor muscles support your bladder and internal organs sufficiently?

The tests here are just about awareness. We cover some simple exercises on the abdominal and pelvic floor muscles later, but for now, I want you to feel where we are talking about.

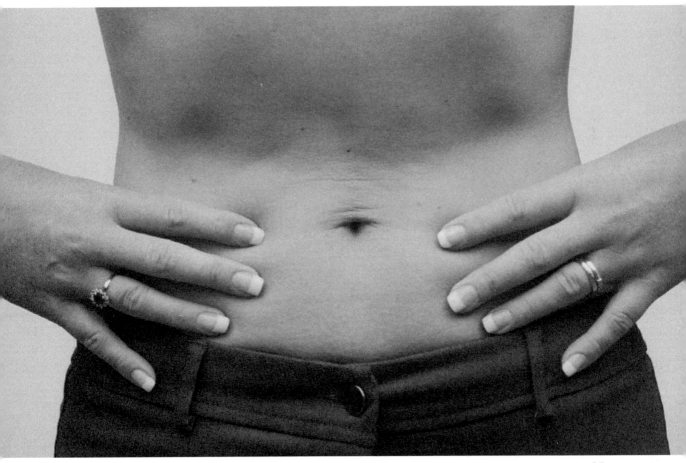

Abdominal muscles

These are key muscles in the posture workout. If you push them with your fingers as you are sitting, they will be relaxed and switched off. Sitting for much of your day in a relaxed state does not help them to be toned, or to look and feel how you probably want them to be. We all know that these muscles look unattractive when they are not toned, but the health benefits of strong, supportive abdominal muscles for control of your low back cannot be underestimated.

> *Place your hands on either side of your waist, fingers on your tummy, and give a good cough. Do you feel the tension in your abdominal wall? If you can, then just do the stomach brace without the cough – you have performed an abdominal muscle tightening which will improve its tone and responsiveness. The trick is not to hold your breath, but build up your ability to do this action easily, while you breathe, and even be able to hold it for up to 10 seconds.*

> *Try this over a week and see how good you feel across the front of your tummy. You will actually improve quickly in the first week as the body and mind connect this action, learn it as a new pattern, and then reinforce it.*

Pelvic floor muscles

The pelvic floor muscles make up the base of your whole body and the platform for your posture. If these muscles are not working well, when you exercise there is often evidence of this for all to see. Pelvic floor weakness is very common and can cause involuntary leaking from the bladder. The small group of muscles that makes up the pelvic floor is often lagging behind the rest of the muscles in tone and responsiveness. It is important that the sluggishness of these muscles is corrected so they respond much more quickly and adequately to the stresses applied through exercise, sexual activity, general work and play.

Like many women I'm sure you have considered and enjoyed the benefits of walking. But are you one of the many (one in four), who to their horror find themselves damp or wet to the point of actual leaking from their bladders? It comes as a huge shock to most women, but it's worse still if you consider it a normal part of aging or being a woman. Childbirth is the most common cause of damage to the muscles and supporting pelvic structures, so there are a lot of women wearing panty liners as they walk, or modifying their drinking to minimize the chance of embarrassing themselves.

The following is a simple standard test for pelvic floor isolation.

> *While you are urinating, try to stop the flow by tensing your pelvic floor muscles. Try to stop the flow mid-stream or near the end of the stream. Your ability to do this will give you an idea of the strength / tone of your pelvic floor muscles.*

Note: This exercise has long been recommended after childbirth, but today it is not advised to repeatedly stop / start the flow of urine as it "confuses the bladder," which may cause problems such as urgency (an urgent need to go to the toilet).

FITNESS LEVEL AND VARIETY OF ACTIVITY

This test determines whether you are achieving the recommended levels of activity you need to keep healthy. Consider any activities that increase or raise your heart rate. Medical experts have proven that any regular physical activity is good for you. You can benefit from as little as 30 minutes spread across the day. In this physical activity assessment, look at whether you are getting enough changes in position (e.g. from standing, sitting, bending).

Guidelines on movement

View movement as an opportunity, not an inconvenience.

Be active in as many ways as possible.

Put together at least 30 minutes of moderate-intensive physical activity on most days if not all days of the week.

If possible, add some vigorous exercises for extra health and fitness. As a bonus you will be helping to keep your bones strong.

Add power to activity. As you move and rest, flow into and out of your day like a continuous workout that gives you both strong and gentle control of your body. Because you choose to improve your posture it will feel good and be good for you.

MODERATE PHYSICAL ACTIVITY*	TIME SPENT IN MINUTES						
	Mon	**Tue**	**Wed**	**Thur**	**Fri**	**Sat**	**Sun**
Physical activity at work							
Walking briskly							
Housework, e.g. vacuuming							
Cleaning, e.g. scrubbing							
Sports							
Taking the stairs, walking to car							
Shopping till you drop							
Sexual play							
Other							
Total time in minutes							

* A good example of moderate-intensive activity is brisk walking at a pace where talking is comfortable but singing is not.

If your schedule shows you are doing less than the recommended physical activity, you may need to build in some more. The more you do the more you benefit.

Now stop feeling bad because you have no time, no energy and no money to get physical. We are simply talking about movement, so let's get empowered.

Postural fitness

What I call postural fitness is being able to sustain a good body alignment without fatigue, mainly because of two things: the first is that you have a relaxed, easy rhythm in what you do; and second, it helps if your day has a balance and variety in the types of activity you mostly do.

Muscles are toned naturally by activity in a variety of ways, which is difficult if you stand all day, drive all day or sit at a workstation. Joints also respond to exercise that challenges the body through a movement range to keep them supple with minimal pain. As a bonus, activity helps to build strong bones.

You may be achieving fitness naturally with gardening, walking and pushing the vacuum around, but perhaps you are not completely straightening up often enough, or reversing the positions that you mainly do. You will find the power of your posture is an "awareness," a feeling of adding quality to your movements.

With the insight this book has given you so far, complete the following:

	POOR	AVERAGE	GOOD	AWESOME
My basic posture in standing is:				
The strength of my abdominals is:				
The strength of my pelvic floor muscles is:				
My level of activity is:				
My postural fitness is:				
I personally rate my posture as:				
Poor: Embarrassed, I know I need to work on this area				
Average: So-so, I feel I could improve				
Good: Quite pleased, I passed the challenges but want to improve				
Awesome: Proud, I could write the book				

If you rate yourself average to poor and/or you are worried about an injury, or suffer from pain, you could go straight to chapter 8, which has special sections designed to help areas of your body that challenge and concern you. Make sure you check this section out if you know you could improve your bladder control and need pelvic floor muscle training.

If you rate yourself average, there are probably areas where you know you could improve, e.g. you may have occasional leakage of urine with coughing, sneezing and laughing though you don't wear pads for playing volleyball – yet!

You may rate yourself as good because you are reasonably fit, walk three or four times per week, and your job and lifestyle offer reasonable variety. Well done. The question and the real challenge is: how will you feel in 10 or 20 or more years? You don't want to become a round-shouldered, leaky little old lady!

If you are awesome in each of these assessments you should be fit, strong and have enough variety in your day to keep you supple – go for your dreams and give this book to someone along the way who needs it.

For most of us, let's continue on and find out why I call good posture "the ultimate exercise."

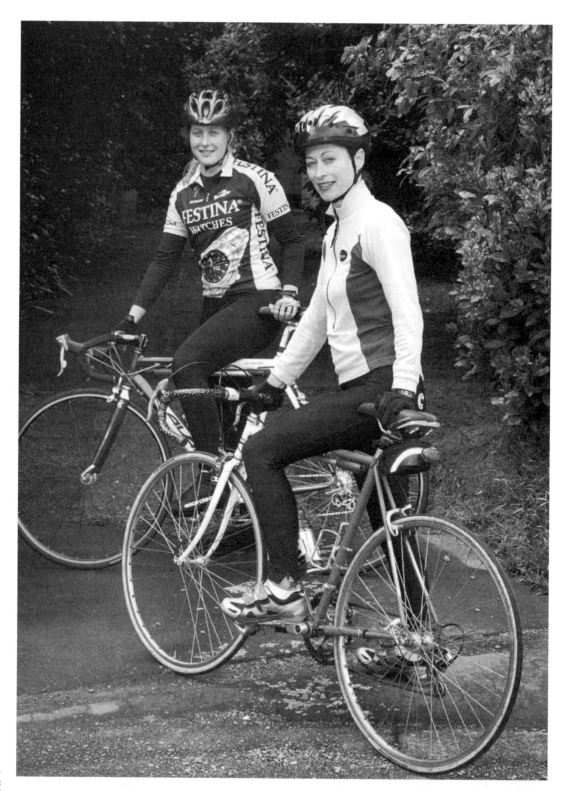

Chapter 4

POSTURE ON THE MOVE

STANDING POWER

If you were a puppet on a string, and I was about to cut off those strings, the best place to hold you to keep you upright would be around your hips and pelvis. Standing strongly comes from gaining power within your torso and pelvic platform. Many disciplines including ballet, sports and martial arts focus on the strength and power of this lower abdominal region.

A ballet teacher who has been teaching her art for over 40 years described to me how she teaches young girls and young women to stand: "I tell the girls to be as long as they can from their hip bones to their rib bones, to widen this gap in their middle. Then I teach them to imagine it is just like trying to zip up a tight pair of jeans, ZIP, then to stop them all hunching up their shoulders and sucking in from their rib cage, I tell them to ZAP or pull down their back side; this gives them a stable pelvis."

This teacher tells the girls that it is important to have their sternum (breast-bone) over their toes, as this suggests a feeling of movement and momentum rather than sitting back and waiting. She believes in the natural beauty of being a woman, that the curves are important, so she emphasizes that the spine is not held rigid and stiff but poised so you are always on balance.

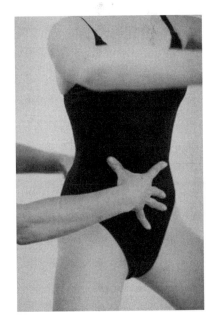

To stand efficiently, the abdominal muscles, low back and pelvic floor muscles work in harmony to maintain a neutral position. You want your lower torso region to be the central focus of your postural control. Too often we find ourselves slouching, standing on one leg leaning our hip out, or just sagging to give our muscles a break – though in fact this is tiring. Ideally, when you get tired you should walk and move out of a standing postition, but if standing is what you need to do, instead of a change of position into a sag, slouch or poor resting stance, pull up with your pelvic floor muscles and brace your lower abdominals – remember the tummy muscle assessment where you coughed and braced to find your deep tummy muscles (see page 36). This should be done while continuing to breathe normally.

Imagine your bony pelvis is like a basin or funnel positioned ever-so-slightly tilted forward but not enough to allow any water to spill out. You can then tilt it either forward or backward but at all times with firm control. Your butt should not poke out or be flattened under, but be somewhere in between these two postures. Perhaps do one, then the other to feel your neutral position. It is important to feel that you can lift your pelvis with your spine and chest, as though a string is pulling you up from the center of your head. This will allow you to keep your spine curved as it should be, and your butt just right.

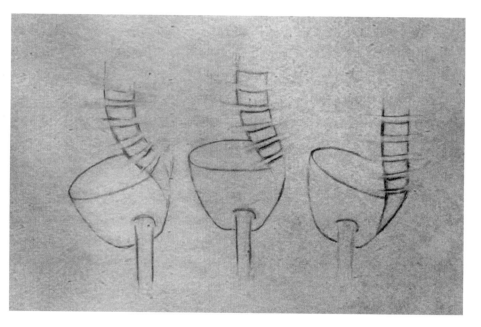

Try to make your tummy muscles do the work here. Do not bend your knees or tuck too much from your spine. Pull in and hold the basin almost level. Health professionals would call this a pelvic tilt exercise, but I don't want you to tilt the pelvis too hard or else you will lose the curve or arch in the small of your back.

Use the front and lower tummy to pull your belly in and keep the internal structures firm. Remember, at this stage the breath must not be held or come from your upper chest; just breathe normally.

If you stand at rest, waiting in a line perhaps, without thinking about it too hard stand with a quality that is similar to a graceful movement. If you stand passively and sag, you will very quickly place strain on your body that can stretch all kinds of tissues, which will then ache either at the time or later. Do you get home from standing at work all day, sit down, put your feet up and think, "Why am I so tired and achy, when I haven't done anything all day?" If so, you need to take an interest in how you are standing. If it is your predominant posture, focus on standing well and practice this till you have it down to an art form. Making a conscious effort to stand well makes your body more responsive to stimuli because you have it switched on. You will love the feeling of power it generates within you.

Ideal standing alignment

Head level, eyes level.

Chest firm.

Tips of shoulders in the same line as your ears.

Tummy held firm.

Pelvic basin tipped more to back than front.

Weight evenly balanced through legs.

Weight evenly on the pads of toes and through heels.

Arches of feet pulled up.

Knees straight but relaxed.

Standing micromoves (mini movements)

Alternate feet and ankle raises up onto the pads of toes and back down.

Pelvic tilt (see page 123) or rock to stretch lower back.

Stand with one leg on slightly raised stool / shelf to relax pelvis.

Stretch quadriceps / hamstrings (see stretching exercises 26 and 27, pages 104 and 107).

Stretch calf muscles (see exercise 28, page 109) to stimulate circulation by increasing the blood flow through these muscles.

Raise and flatten arches of feet.

Forward bend at hips to stretch hamstrings and low back.

Round and arch back to alter spinal curves.

Just for fun

Do the occasional pirouette.

Stand in a plié or half-squat position for a minute to strengthen quads.

Think about something really, really funny.

Stand on one leg for 30 seconds to stimulate balance.

Stand on tiptoes for 30 seconds.

Remember: Standing power is in your muscles rather than your spine bones. I do not wish you to flatten out your low back curve. It's more a belly-in maneuver than a spinal curve flattening.

Walking power

Many women discover the power of posture as they walk. Your trunk should remain essentially still and your arms and legs should propel you forward. The plumb line from the side view can be vertical or slightly inclined forward if you wish to increase your pace.

We all have seen images of native women (and men) carrying loads on their heads gracefully and effortlessly, suggesting an innate control. How can they do that?

The spine is designed to withstand compressive loads, so this enables us to do activities such as land safely from a jump off a high wall, or jump up and down without crushing or damaging our spinal bones. People can hold large weights on their heads because we are cushioned by discs in between our vertebrae and have muscles acting as guy-wires, holding us balanced.

We all have the ability to walk well and some women seem to have effortless grace and beauty; this is not about forcing a quality of controlled posture, but about owning the feeling. Be proud of yourself out there, walking your body positively. If you have ever tried yoga you will know that part of its simplicity is to appreciate and value the movement or posture, to feel how you are placing your body.

So, yoga while you walk! Can you do that? Try it.

Lift your neck up and out, look directly forward, breathe gently and deeply, and hold your spine with your back muscles.

Think tall, imagine a piece of string pulling you up from your head, not to straighten all your spinal curves but just to elongate your muscles.

Push your arms forward, aiming for in front of your sternum / breast bone.

Lift out of your pelvis and step with your heel first, then land and push off through your toes.

You will feel and look really beautiful, anywhere, anytime.

Ideal walking alignment

Head and eyes level.

Tuck chin in, with ears in line with shoulders.

Keep chest firmly forward but not stuck out.

Tummy actively pulled in.

Spinal curves neutral, as for standing.

Pelvis / hip bones pretty much level.

Heel / toe action as you walk.

Take even strides.

Think about having fluidity of movement, i.e. think graceful movements.

Walking micromoves

Walk faster by using the momentum of your arms swinging more quickly.

Push forward to a central spot in front of your tummy.

Pull in your pelvic floor as you walk, try to hold for 10 seconds while continuing to breathe normally.

Think: gliding "Zen-like" as you walk.

Alternate walking pace from rapid to slow at intervals.

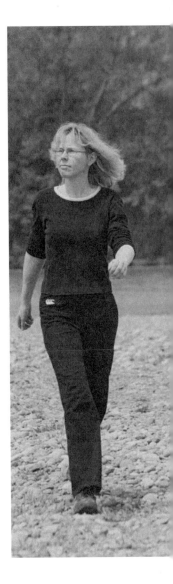

Just for fun

Smile or wink at everyone you walk past.

Walk barefoot over sand.

Walk through the water at the beach or river's edge to stimulate proprioception (this is a term to describe "how it feels for you").

Walk slowly and talk.

Get a dog ...

POWER IN JOGGING, RUNNING, SPRINTING

The same posture for walking (torso firm, pump the arms and legs) can be applied when you jog, or if you wish to increase your pace. Your upper body should remain constant, both upright and aligned with good spinal curves. Your head and neck should be level and there should be minimal wobbling of your body. As your arms and legs pump harder, there should be no extra effort seen.

For extra speed, the plumb line can be inclined slightly further forward. To feel where this is, keep your body straight, rise up on your toes and tip forward to where you feel you are almost about to fall, then step out of it. Do this a few times till you feel the position. This is the optimal position to run fast.

SITTING POWER

If you took a simple kitchen chair and asked ten people to sit on it, you would probably see ten different positions, such as perching on the chair's edge, curved in a "C" shape (butt right at the edge, legs outstretched, head and neck poked forward). Some people will push their back well into the chair, erect and supported. Perhaps some would sit sideways. Have you seen people turn a chair around and sit straddled with their arms leaning on the back of the chair? And then there is the leaning-forward, elbows-on-knees, cup-chin-in-hands posture. Each posture conveys a different message, places your body in different proportions of risk to the spine and will tire you to different degrees if you stay in it for a period of time.

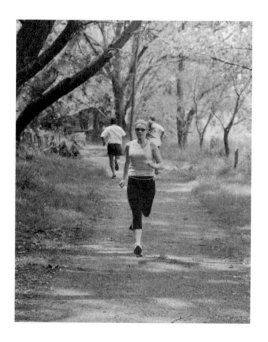

Feel how to sit correctly

Sit in a simple kitchen chair or office chair, over-sway your back and really feel an arched, sway-back posture. Then move the other way, round into a ball. Somewhere between the two extremes, just a little forward (swayed forward) of neutral is good lumbar (low back) spinal alignment.

The trick in sitting is to maintain the spinal curves in exactly the same position as when standing in good alignment, to adopt a position that suits the activity and not stay in one position for too long, but move your body every 20 minutes or so. As soon as you lose the ability to maintain an ideal position, get up and move any way you want to. Try to loosen up the kinks and be nice to your body, and it will be nice back. This would be a good time to do spontaneous stretching (see page 70).

Sitting at a workstation might be your predominant work posture. Think about the load your spine is handling as you do this. There is actually more body weight on your spine than if you were standing. The ideal "sitting-back-in-the-seat" posture that places the spinal curves in a position supported by the chair back is the most appropriate (providing that you actually use the seat back for support and not lean away from it).

After gardening for a few hours, to come in and sit front-to-back on a straight chair, or lean forward and place your elbows on your knees would naturally stretch your low back out and would be relaxing, feel good, and be quite suitable.

If you were waiting for an interview, or were in a meeting, you may project a dynamic personality if you were alert and upright on the edge of your chair. When sitting in a café with friends your posture radiates your natural poise. It conveys how you are feeling about yourself and others around you.

Whatever way you sit, how do you keep those curves in line? It's in the way you handle your body. Sit strongly rather than passively, which will result in sagging. This gives your muscles the power and support over the joints and ligaments by adopting and feeling good alignment. Again, having good firm abdominal and pelvic floor muscles helps to achieve this form.

Sitting posture check

> *Head neutral, eyes level.*
>
> *Ears in line with shoulders.*
>
> *Shoulders slightly back.*
>
> *Breasts forward (no, not jutting out, just elevated).*
>
> *Tummy held in.*
>
> *Sit on butt bones, thighs level, butt right back in seat.*
>
> *Feet flat on floor.*
>
> *Knees at right angles.*

SITTING AT WORKSTATION

Sitting for most of the day is tiring on the spine and, as muscles very quickly protest at being held in one position, you will often find you end up slouching over your desk. It is important to have the correct seating and setup of your workstation and to understand how to benefit from it. Back supports in a chair are great providing you sit back into them as you use your keyboard or write. Too often people use stretching movements, reaching to answer the phone or use the mouse, and are not supported at all by their chair.

The ideal sitting posture at a workstation allows you to be relaxed and supported with no reaching or loading of your body in odd or prolonged positions. A good thing to remember is to have your feet flat on the floor or supported on a footstool to keep your hips and knees bent to 90 degrees. And remember, the home setup is as important as the one at the office.

Ideal sitting alignment at workstation

Low back curve supported and relaxed.

Head in line with shoulders.

Chin slightly tucked in.

Shoulders level and pulled back and down, relaxed with no tension.

Breathing even and gentle.

Legs horizontal, feet flat on floor or stool.

Legs not crossed.

When reaching forward, ideally do it from your hip level. Make your tummy muscles work to pull your torso forward and keep yourself aligned with your spinal curves just as they are. Do not bend from either the base of neck or from about bra level as this causes a strain on your body.

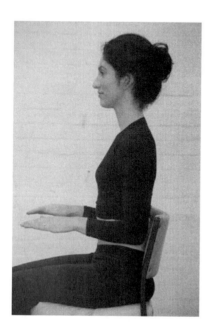

RELAXED SITTING

Maintain low back curve.

Sit on buttock bones.

Let tension go with deep relaxed breathing.

Just for fun.

Turn a chair around and sit backwards.

Sit cross-legged.

Sit on the floor.

Sit sidesaddle on a table.

LIFTING

For professional, trained Olympic weightlifters their whole center of being is geared towards lifting, and they have to do it properly, with control, but they all have their individual styles. What is the secret they share? The lumbar curve is maintained throughout the whole lift. Here is how you can adopt the way they lift, without the tight leotards.

Ideal lifting technique

Lean shoulders slightly forward, simultaneously sticking butt out.

Bend knees, keeping heels flat on the floor for stability.

Keep eyes level and focus on strong abdominal control.

Bend to 90 degrees, grasp object to be lifted, then drive up with legs and butt.

Do not hold breath.

Do not reach across or out from your body for the object you are lifting.

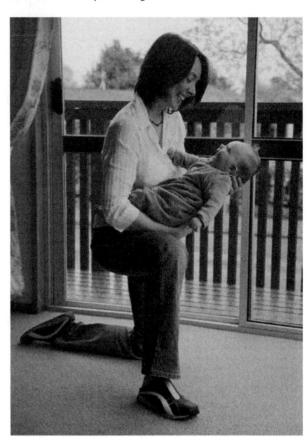

When you lift off the floor you increase your low back injury risk by 75%, so this has to be done with a deep squat, wrapping your arms around the object you wish to lift, keeping it close to your body.

If the object is light, such as a golf ball you want to retrieve out of a hole, you can also hurt your back because you tend not to think about technique – you lean forward, often twisting your spine, and overall do not take it seriously. So it is ideal to raise one leg, lean on the golf club and bend to retrieve the ball.

When lifting a heavy object you will usually remember good technique, but around the home, the everyday thoughtless lifting of shopping bags out of the car, the vacuum cleaner off the floor into the closet, and the baby into the bassinet causes most incidences of back pain. Keeping in good postural shape can greatly reduce the incidence of low back pain by keeping your body flexible, strong and fit.

If you have just had a baby, lifting is an activity that you will be doing more and more of. The hormonal influence on your body means all your ligaments will be softer and stretchier, and women often find they ache from the demands that a new baby places on the household, so good posture is especially important.

Remember: If you cannot lift safely – don't. (Did you know that it's okay to ask for help?)

Taking a break

Look for and remember to take the natural breaks in your tasks, which you may know as micropauses (no, they are not just for typing). I call these natural movement releases micromoves, because they are still a form of activity.

A variety of movements gives a natural rhythm to your day, and helps you to keep working longer without injury.

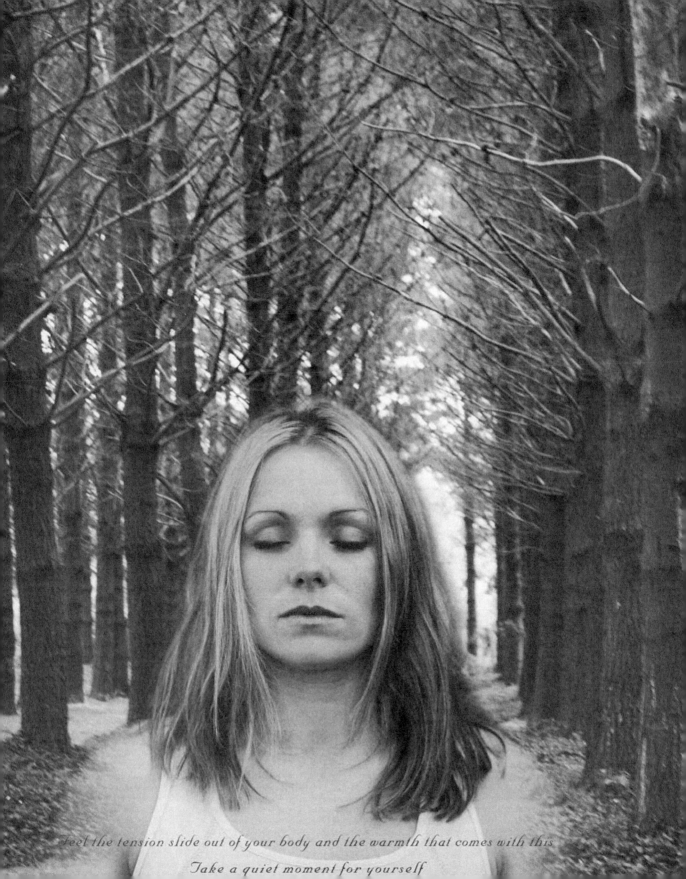

feel the tension slide out of your body and the warmth that comes with this

Take a quiet moment for yourself

Chapter 5

Posture at rest

Breathing

A no-stress, no-tension, calm body is a joy. Part of this joy is the beautiful paradox of breathing, both powerful and wonderful in arousal, and gentle and deep with relaxation. Breathing well is a blend of both relaxation and awareness.

By using your breathing positively and powerfully, you gain a personal insight into how you are doing each day, and monitor how you are feeling. Your breathing can be really useful to get the mind and body connecting with each other. Breathing is the key to gaining control of your tension, your fears – and even your childbirth! The art of breathing is to not let anyone know you are doing it and having such a good time. Breathing is an art form; it requires you to practice letting go, and learning to be at peace with the world. Think: in through your nose (inhale), out through your mouth (exhale).

Feel how to breathe well

Place your hands on your upper tummy, one above the other, just below your breasts. Breathe in so that only your lower hand rises, and then let go. This is belly breathing, or deep breathing. Do it about three times, then relax.

Slow deep breathing is probably the single best anti-stress medicine we have. When you bring air down into the lungs, where oxygen exchange is most efficient, everything changes. Heart rate slows, blood pressure decreases, muscles relax, anxiety ceases and the mind clears. Breathing helps to oxygenate your blood and remove the waste products.

THE BREATHING MUSCLE

Unconsciously and consciously, the diaphragm is the key breathing muscle. When efficiently working, it draws the lungs down and out, creates effective breathing, and allows voice control, as in singing. The diaphragm is a key muscle for releasing tension and stress (and also a key control for intra-abdominal pressure when lifting). It needs to work in harmony with the tummy and pelvic floor muscles, not against them.

Deep breathing for relaxation

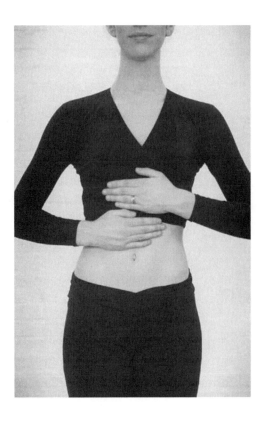

> *Smooth out face, calm your mind.*
>
> *Close eyes (optional).*
>
> *Open chest position by pulling shoulders back and down.*
>
> *Shoulders relaxed and down as you breathe.*
>
> *Keep mouth relaxed.*
>
> *Breathe in through nose, breathe out through mouth.*
>
> *Breathe in slowly over 5 seconds, out over same count.*
>
> *Do 3 to 5 breaths in one set, take a moment, then do another set.*
>
> *Perform this type of breathing throughout the day.*

Breathing is a big help to relax our bodies and focus and concentrate on tasks. It is a great micromove to perform good, deep breaths to oxygenate our bodies and remove waste products. If you practice yoga or meditation then you will have been instructed in the art of deep breathing and will already understand and enjoy the "feel good" of gentle breathing exercises.

BREATHING EXERCISES

Everybody benefits from breathing and relaxation techniques, whether you are an elite athlete about to perform, are organizing a kid's birthday party where chaos rules, feeling overtired and generally fatigued or just feeling unsure what to do next. Some medical conditions (e.g. asthma, respiratory disease or a heart problem) and certain medications may cause your body to idle too fast, generating inner stress and overworking your "engine."

In some cases, the only time a woman may have had any instruction on breathing or relaxation advice is in labor when breathing focus is a controlling, calming influence and is used as a natural form of pain relief. It is generally considered today that women need to do whatever they feel they need to for their labor such as walking around and changing postures, and so breathing is less emphasized. It will be actively encouraged when or if they need to gain control of the pain through stages of their labor. In the second stage of labor, when the baby's head is crowning, the midwife or doctor may coach the woman to pant in short shallow breaths, to try to slow down uncontrolled pushing where tearing the perineum or pelvic floor muscles is a risk.

So chances are, you have never been encouraged to develop good breathing as a focus for relaxation and centring yourself.

We don't always breathe correctly, naturally. It would be nice if we could simply breathe correctly and not think about how we do it but, with our lives becoming much busier and more stressful, sometimes it is useful to understand the benefits of slow, gentle breathing. It is a good idea not to hold your breath if you are straining your body such as with lifting or pushing; and do not do episodes of rapid, short shallow breathing except for a very short time. With every energetic burst of activity we need to breathe appropriately.

Athletes expel their breath when they hit a ball or lift a weight, so they direct their energy correctly. They sometimes have to learn to do this and you may find that tightening muscles, such as when you lift, without holding your breath is very difficult to achieve. Let's test you:

Tighten the tummy muscles – go, grip and squeeze. Did you hold your breath or suck in your tummy? You should ideally be able to tense any muscle, such as the tummy or the pelvic floor muscles, while you breathe in and out, smile, look cool …

Try again. This time, maintain your breathing in and out, grip with your tummy muscles but not give any sign that you are doing it, so that you use maximum work with minimal effort.

Subjecting ourselves to stress in our lives causes muscles to tense and our breathing rate to quicken. It's like keeping your foot on the accelerator while you are waiting at the lights, keeping the engine revving, which, my husband says knowingly, increases wear and tear on the motor, puts pressure on the brakes and other systems in the car and uses the fuel too fast.

Breathing rates vary from 9 to 12 breaths per minute. Check for a minute and see if you are in this range. If you find your breathing pattern is fast, go and get some advice from a health professional. Panic attacks or anxiety attacks are more and more common today. Coping with an increase in stress in our lives often means we automatically hold our breath or breathe quickly or too much with the top of our lungs. We can do this in short bursts, but if we are under constant pressure and maintain this type of breathing we may develop symptoms of exhaustion, dizziness and feeling unwell. If you suffer from these conditions they respond well to good breathing management. It is a key self-treatment strategy, which gives control to these symptoms naturally.

In fact, your ability to experience gentle deep breathing is a secret weapon giving control of your body in every situation and posture. You can consciously use your breathing when you do any of the positions and exercises that you move through in your day.

RELAXATION

Throughout time people have always found ways to relax and cleanse the inner self, such as sauna baths followed by flagellation with birch switches; yoga and meditation; massage and fasting techniques. In order to be healthy and happy, relaxation is as important as exercise. It is like night to day, up to down, sleeping to being awake.

Once you are breathing well there are many ways to further reduce the tension in your body and you need to invest some of your time in doing nothing! But relaxation is more than just doing nothing. Relaxation is a special space you create to care for yourself, or to reenergize yourself.

Steps to relaxation

Imagine your whole body "heavy and warm."

Then allow your mind to focus on different parts of your body and let the tension go progressively out of each part of your body.

Imagine a beautiful place you can visit – go there in your mind.

Make the atmosphere relaxing – soft light, music and warmth is good.

Make an ESPS moment (see below).

Breathe with belly breathing.

Try micromoves (see pages 110–111).

ESPS MOMENTS

Take a moment ... an ESPS (emotional, spiritual, physical and social) moment.

Women today seem to have more difficulty trying to balance all the many aspects of their lives. Some superwomen are already on it, but for the rest of us, whew, we can barely get up in the morning. I wish you to consider that getting harmony into your life is in the way you balance the physical, emotional, social and spiritual aspects. This is about what you do, what you feel, what you share and what you value. I call this an ESPS moment. Try to make an ESPS moment each day.

Achieving internal as well as external balance is what improving your posture is all about. Sometimes you may take a moment for yourself when you take a coffee break, go for a walk, or stop the car at the beach; an ESPS moment is that same feeling, transferred to the office or home at any time on an ordinary day.

For example, next time you go for a walk – when you go to collect the mail or walk across the office:

Lift up out of your pelvis by lengthening up from your hip bones to your rib bones (do it).

Imagine an urn on your head like a weight you need to balance, hold your trunk steady while you move your arms and legs (feel it).

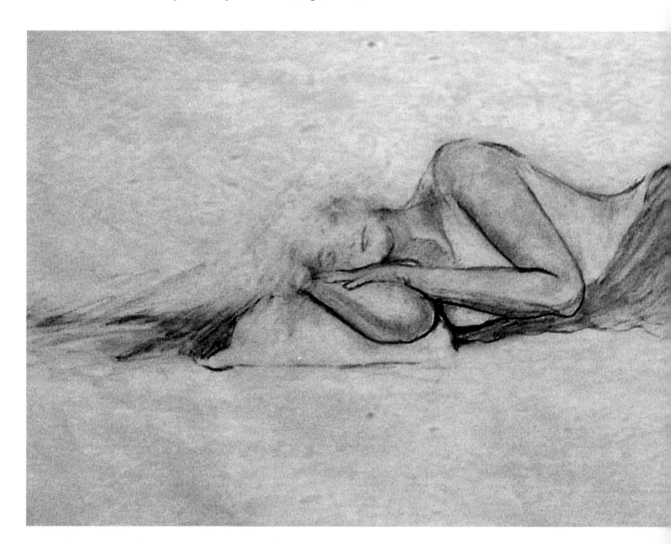

Smile from the inside (share it).

Breathe deeply and gently and enjoy the atmosphere (value it).

SLEEPING

A restful and rejuvenating night's sleep is bliss. The positions that you sleep in may affect how you feel in the morning – refreshed and invigorated or stiff and slow to get moving. The mattress and pillows are also a significant factor in creating comfortable sleep. You certainly know about it when you sleep on the wrong pillow and wake up with a sore neck, a headache, and feel tired all day. Then there are

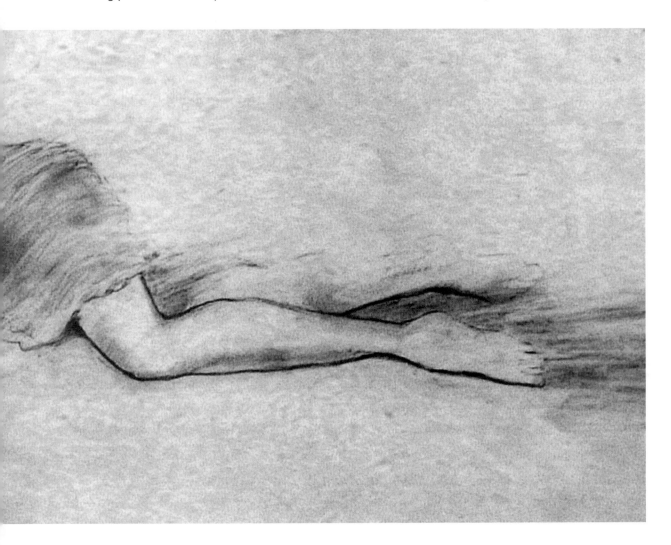

the psychological and social factors that can impact how you sleep, such as stresses that worry you, your partner tossing and turning beside you, children who come to visit in the middle of the night, the wrong phone number that wakes you, or the cats fighting next door!

To ensure a comfortable posture for sleeping, think about what position you actually prefer to lie in. If you sleep on your side, the space between your head and the mattress is wider than if you are on your back so it makes sense to use one and a half pillows to support your neck in this space – the half pillow being a soft, moldable, punch-into-shape one that stays in place, so you can curl it into the gap at the base of your neck and support your neck. If you can find suitable pillows try to take them with you when you sleep away from home, especially if you have a neck problem. If you are sleeping away from home, a rolled-up soft towel placed lengthways in the base of the pillowcase can support your neck curve and suffice.

Modern pillows are often one piece of hard foam that bounces your head and lacks the "moldability" to your neck. So choose a firm, moldable, retainable-shaped pillow that will support the curve of your neck. If you have lots of pillows for decoration, try not to sleep with them all at the back of your neck. They will stop your spine from being restored into a neutral resting position and will probably make you restless through the night. Similarly, a reading pillow can be a cause of poor posture in bed, and should only be used for short periods of time and not for sleeping since it sags you into too much of a C-shaped curve.

If you do like to lie on your side, and your back gets stiff when you wake, try tucking a pillow underneath your top leg to stop your spine from twisting or rotating into positions that can make you stiff in the morning. Check that your sleeping surface is not too soft.

If you sleep on your back or tummy you only need one smaller pillow. Try one under your knees to relax your low back curve – having two pillows doesn't mean both have to be under your head, rounding your spine.

Many people sleep on their tummy, one leg bent up, head turned to one side. The main potential problem with this position is that your neck is held in a turned position. You should be careful if you have a neck problem, but if you don't, the spine is actually relaxed and in a fairly neutral shape and can be quite comfortable.

In researching sleeping postures, I was interested to note that some tribal people of Africa sleep on the ground with an ear against the dirt, a hand tucked under their neck and no mat at all, so they can listen for the rumble of wild animals. It is thought that these tribal people naturally keep their spines in good shape while they sleep on the hard ground because the ribs gently move the spine up and down as they breathe, moving their joints. Himalayan people can sleep curled up in a ball on all fours huddled against the cold, perched on the side of a mountain in freezing conditions. For the majority of us, outdoor sleeping makes us long for our bed at home, which suddenly seems really comfortable. Today beds are firm but supportive and kinder to the "bony" parts of us compared with the ground. There is a wide range of different sleeping surfaces and prices today; in choosing a bed that fits you can be like Goldilocks. While going back to sleeping on the floor is extreme, be fussy about the type of mattress and surface you do sleep on and find one that supports and suits you.

Good sleep hygiene can be described as a "ritual that induces good, productive sleep," and you may like to get into the habit of doing some or all of these before you go to bed:

Aids to restful sleep

> *Take a warm bath.*
>
> *Have a warm milky drink.*
>
> *Think all your thoughts before you get into bed.*
>
> *Use bed to sleep, NOT to do all your bills.*
>
> *Make it soft, peaceful and dreamy in your bedroom.*
>
> *Have a notepad and pen handy for all those critical points you remember or dream up in the middle of the night. Jot them down so you can let your mind turn off.*

There is a time for exciting, zipping-around-in-your-head thoughts, such as thinking about all tomorrow's activities, what you didn't get done today ... but maybe this should be done when you are out walking or by turning the TV off a few minutes early. Have all that thinking out of the way before bedtime.

Encouraging good habits for your body to relax before you try to sleep allows you to unwind and destress *before* you get into bed. By avoiding stimulants or complicated thoughts at bedtime you will also enhance a good night's sleep.

Chapter 6

POSTURE AND SEXUALITY

If you want to think of a perfect example of a body in action and relaxation, with all its grace and beauty, richness and fullness – think about making love.

This chapter examines the uniquely feminine aspect of posture which involves the area from the base of your torso – the pelvic floor platform – and the sexuality component of body movement. To fully express herself a woman should be aware of and enjoy her sexuality. Women have known this for centuries. Think about Middle Eastern belly dancing: the way to do a belly dance well is to imagine you are gripping a pencil with your vaginal muscles and drawing a circle with the pencil. As you become more expert you draw the body and wings of a butterfly. What a clever and subtle way to exercise your pelvic floor muscles.

The key to your sexuality is part of the same key to your posture. By using body awareness in yourself, breathing to heighten pleasure and to calm, and increasing the tone of your pelvic floor muscles, you will improve sensitivity and increase your response to stimuli. Exercise therapy is an easy and effective way to improve pelvic floor muscle tone and the advantages are both physical and sexual:

- improvement in orgastic function (a fancy term for the ability to achieve orgasm)
- an increase in support for internal organs
- added protection to low back from injury in lifting and straining
- strength and control over urinary leakage, urgency and prolapse

If you have missed out on pelvic floor exercise education there is much to know. In some cultures, women are taught the importance and value of control over their pelvic floor muscles for sexual enhancement. Pelvic floor training is repetitive, selective voluntary contraction and relaxation of specific pelvic floor muscles.

A toned muscle feels better, works better and generally has less go wrong with it. So the same training that you put into other areas of your body can be applied to the pelvic floor.

Pelvic floor muscles

There is nothing between your lower internal organs and the floor except your pelvic floor muscles (perineum). These small, hidden muscles and other supportive structures such as ligaments and a kind of woven tissue called fascia have a very important role in keeping your insides where they should be. The pelvic floor muscles are a rival force to your diaphragm as they both get tightened as you cough, lift, laugh and so on.

You need to work the inside muscles of your body just as you work the outside muscles, trying to get them really strong and responsive. These muscles are an integral part of your posture and knowing more about them is very important for all women, young or old.

The pelvic floor is a muscular sling with three openings (sphincters) for your bladder, vagina and bowel. This muscle group has major functions for women, keeping their bladders watertight and their internal

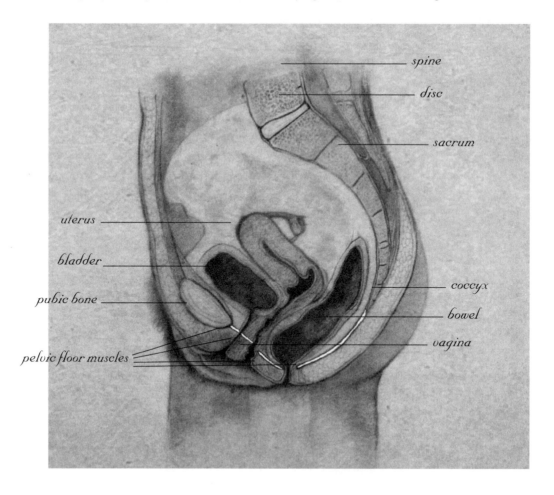

organs supported during pregnancy and throughout life. The muscles must stretch for birth, often getting cut or torn in the process, and don't always bounce back into shape after childbirth naturally, sometimes taking a year to recover. They are influenced by hormonal changes in the menstual cycle and menopause and are intimately involved in the sexual arousal response.

It is important for most women and their partners to be sexually responsive, that is, to identify and be in touch with sexual feelings, to play an active role in and enjoy sex. A benefit of an increase in pelvic floor muscle tone is to heighten the potential for sexual pleasure.

So how do you train pelvic floor muscles?

The art of pelvic floor exercises is in appreciating two actions (see page 76). Start with the first action, especially if you have just had a baby or are recovering from surgery. It is important to really identify and feel this action and be confident of knowing you are doing it correctly before doing the second action. I am sure you will enjoy doing these exercises and after successfully learning both, use a blend of the two over the rest of your life.

When first learning how to do them, you will sometimes feel a little achy in the lower tummy, usually just because you are trying too hard. So do not work too hard, but allow yourself to appreciate the sensations of internal power and control and have lots of little rests in between as you go.

SEXUAL EXPRESSION

With or without a partner, the ultimate best time to practice pelvic floor exercises has to be with sexual expression. As you master pelvic floor exercises there will be positive benefits for more than just you. With sexual play it can be quite fun, and we in the therapy business call it biofeedback. By communicating with your partner, with penetration you can both feel the response to your exercise efforts.

Try quick flicks (the first action) to rapidly "squeeze and try to slice your partner into little pieces." Then with the second action, tell your partner, "I'm going to squeeze you and slow you as you try to withdraw." This can be a real challenge because it is so hard to concentrate!

Developing toned pelvic floor muscles can be great for your sex life, but it takes the whole of our bodies to really make the sexual arousal response complete and fulfilling. Sexual enjoyment is more than just about achieving orgasms, it is more like an ESPS moment – an emotional, social, physical and spiritual connection – for both women and men, especially as we get older. A myth that has confused a lot of men and women for years is that vaginal orgasms are the true female orgasm response. While the vaginal (pelvic floor) muscles are certainly involved by involuntarily contracting at the end of the response (which is one reason I suggest you tone the pelvic floor muscles as much as possible), overwhelmingly the climactic trigger for most women is to have direct or indirect stimulation of the clitoris.

POSTURE AND POSITIONING

To explore a full and satisfying sexual experience, your posture and positioning can increase or decrease the sensation to the clitoris.

Try a posture where you are able to position your clitoris against your man's pubic bone or symphysis pubis. What is this? Press on your own pubic area and feel the front of your pelvic bone. This is a hard bony platform that men also have on the front of their pelvis. Couples can position the woman so she can stimulate her clitoris against this bone of her partner.

Where the woman is on top, the secret is to rock forward and backward against the bone rather than slide up and down the shaft of the penis. This movement is a pelvic tilt or pelvic rock movement, tucking your butt under and back out, rolling to suit the stimulation you give yourself. In the missionary position, place pillows under your hips and encourage your partner to do the pelvic tilt action which will

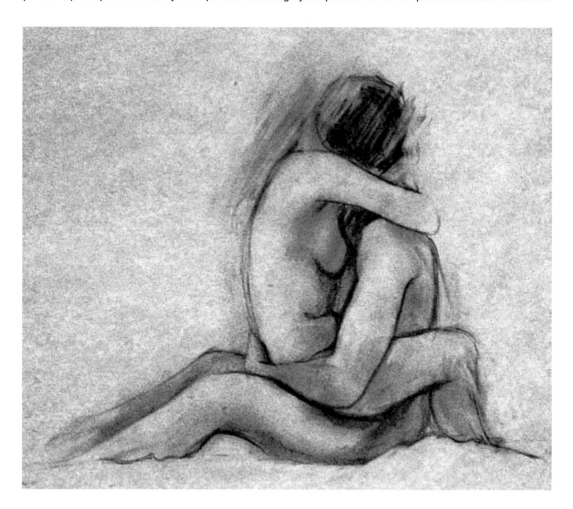

satisfy him while allowing you to receive maximum stimulation on your clitoris.

The positions where partners face each other, such as where the woman is on top, have the advantage of stimulating the G spot or spots, positioned on the front vaginal wall up about the length of your half-curled-in fingers. This obscure place inside a woman is up under the pubic bone and seems to be connected closely with the urethra or bladder tube. Women describe a feeling of wanting to empty their bladder when pressed on this spot. Similar spots can be found in more than one point within the vagina. Stimulating the area with two fingers is usually enough pressure to allow an orgasm to happen. Gentle finger pressure in a variety of ways can be the easiest for both parties.

Anne Hooper states in her book, *The Kama Sutra*, that ancient positions in sexual intercourse were designed with the aim of increasing sexual tension, and by building up the tension in the vaginal muscles a woman can experience a more intense orgasm when that tension is explosively relieved. Anne Hooper describes three positions where a woman can enhance her pelvic floor strengthening.

Mare's position: "This technique can be applied to enhance a number of positions. In it, the woman uses her vaginal muscles to squeeze the penis. This arouses pelvic sensuality for both him and her. Experimentation with different positions will reveal which one the vaginal squeeze works with effectively. For many people, the best is the man-on-top clasping position (missionary position), but others find it enjoyable where the woman sits astride the man, either facing him or with her back to him."

Pair of tongs: "With her legs bent at the knee, the woman sits astride, facing the man, who lies flat on his back. She draws his penis inside her and squeezes it repeatedly with her vagina, holding it for a long time. Penetration is deep."

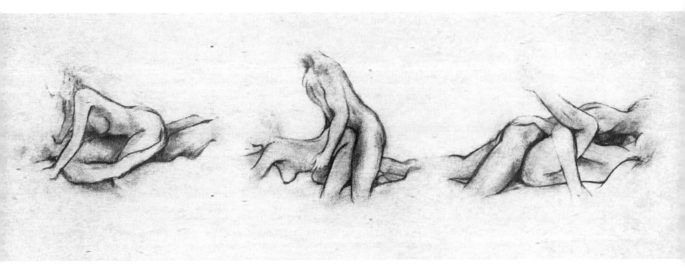

Snake trap: "The woman sits astride the man, facing him, and each partner holds the other's feet. This allows the couple to rock themselves back and forth in a stimulating seesaw-like movement but, since it restricts thrusting, it is best adopted when the man is tired, or is satisfied and is making love again for his partner's pleasure."

I do believe orgasms are great for premenstrual engorgement and pain. As a physiotherapist I know that movement is good for relieving aches and pains. When there is not immediate bruising or bleeding we often apply heat, and that is why some women will use a heat pack on their tummy when they have premenstrual pain. Orgasm actually lifts and moves the uterus and cervix almost 90 degrees upright and increases the blood flow to the pelvic region. What a great way to relieve this congestion and get things moving.

In the privacy of your own space, try self-pleasuring (masturbation) for your own benefit, including for premenstrual ache, but also at other times of the month, whenever you feel the need.

SEXUAL DYSFUNCTION

Some of the problems described by women include lack of sexual interest, inability to experience orgasm, lubrication difficulties, and non-pleasurable sex.

A women's sexuality aura may be affected by many internal and external factors, some of which are:

- menopausal changes – hormonal changes giving rise to a decrease in lubrication, hot flashes and emotional roller coasters including symptoms of depression
- breastfeeding may impact negatively on your arousal due to fatigue and the constant demand that children are making on you
- stress and lack of regular exercise
- hormonal peaks and changes throughout your cycle
- just because – no reason!

Female sexual dysfunction has been said to increase as we get older and enter mid-life. The most recent findings strongly suggest that sexual response declines significantly with aging, and the other parameters of sexual function assessed – libido (frequency of sexual thoughts), frequency of sexual activities, and vaginal dyspareunia (pain) — are differentially affected by the menopausal transition.

Other factors can have an effect at any age. The penis has been shown to boomerang-bend upwards in its shape with intercourse. If the top of the vaginal wall has stretched, this may be a reason you have reduced sensations vaginally with some positions. As the vaginal wall alters shape with arousal and intercourse, the sensations and sensitive regions within the vagina will also change, be different with different partners, alter with babies and surgery, and so sensitive communicating is needed to find the most pleasurable way. Positions where the couples face away, for example where the man is on top and the woman faces down, puts penetration pressure on the back wall or bowel wall of the vagina and therefore there may be a reduction in the internal sensations for women with rectocycele or bowel prolapse or laxity.

Researchers are finding out a lot more about this whole region in terms of sexual dysfunction in women, but all agree that communication increases intimacy and pleasure. Very little progress has been made in understanding sexual function and dysfunction in women, one of the problems being the difficulty in evaluating the emotional and personal distress aspect. This just means we need more data, more information and more women speaking with each other, not just researchers, on this subject in general. When women talk more freely with their partners, the sexual experience can be greatly enhanced.

Good
posture is
the ultimate
exercise. The
postural workout
provides balance
within your body
by bringing
symmetry to your
shape and form to
your function.

If you do this
workout regularly
you will keep your
body supple
and strong.

Chapter 7

THE POSTURE WORKOUT

I describe good posture as the ultimate exercise. To help you to maintain your ability to have good posture over your entire life, I have designed a very specific postural workout that provides balance within your body by bringing symmetry to your shape and form to your function. If you do this workout regularly, say three times a week, you will keep your body supple and strong.

The posture workout is your exercise script, providing tailored exercise from top to toe in an easy, moderate or more difficult form. The workout should be enjoyable and most of the movements are designed to be done as part of your normal day-to-day activity – the exercises can be done with a glass of wine nearby, or during and after you have a walk – and may be continued right through your life.

All bodies need and actually crave a variety of tasks and movements. Exercises really are just regular movements that you do like squats or bicep curls. Breathing deeply and well is exercise, just as activities like walking, gardening, swimming or gym class.

You may participate in a sport that covers all the aspects of a balanced workout, but many sports are repetitive in certain ways and can actually lead to imbalance. This is why the posture workout is so important. It will help keep you free of aches and pains and will correct all the unnatural movements, such as bending in one direction (usually forward and twisted), sitting too long, lifting too much or rotating too often in your day.

The workout involves:

- Stretching your body, both spontaneously, as a cat will stretch when it wakes up (this is just like a yawn for your body), and more seriously, such as warming up and down in a workout. Stretching will keep your movements fluid, your body supple and free of pain.
- Strengthening exercises, which are both static (stationary) and dynamic (moving); these are also highly beneficial to protect yourself from injury and tone your shape.

STRETCHING

Stretching is the way to keep flexibility in both your muscles and your joints. The more your body is held in one position such as sitting at a computer, the more you are at risk of shortening and tightening up your body. This is why you feel tired doing nothing. Some areas of your body have a tendency to stiffen and shorten (for example, the front of the hip from sitting and the chest muscles from working at a keyboard), making good posture more difficult to achieve. If these parts shorten it leads to weakness in the opposing muscles, in this instance your butt/low back from the hip and upper back from the chest, both essential muscles you want to be strong and shapely.

Regular stretching that tones and shapes your body by providing a balance to your muscle groups reduces the time needed to work on strengthening and you can concentrate on just the pure enjoyment of activity such as a brisk walk.

SPONTANEOUS STRETCHING

Stretch anytime, just till you feel tension but not discomfort or pain. Don't worry about a warm-up, the length of hold of the stretch or when you do it – this is a feel-good, stretch-out-the-wrinkles, elongate-the-spine, letting-go movement.

Any of the stretches in the workout can be done spontaneously if you keep your breathing relaxed and take them just to the end of comfort. Think of this more as an anti-stiffness exercise, a regular opposing movement to what you have been doing, and a gentle way of feeling good. For example, after you have been working spread out your arms and stretch your chest, like a big yawn.

SERIOUS STRETCHING

Part of an athlete's training session is warm-up stretching and warm-down stretching. The stretching of muscles and joints gets the body and mind prepared and ready for vigorous and sometimes sudden activity. At rest, blood flow and nutrients to muscles are concentrated in the vital centers: heart, liver and digestive organs. To exercise well, the blood flow needs to be diverted to the exercising muscles and provide lubrication to joints. So it makes sense to do about 10 minutes of warm-up activity before a serious session of stretching. This can be as simple as a walk or some step-ups to kick-start your circulation. Put on warm, comfortable gear, try to increase your heart rate, feel loose mentally.

After this warm-up, aim to stretch slowly and gently to the point of discomfort and hold for about 20 seconds, breathing all through the movement. Do each stretch about three times, at least twice a week, maximum about four times a week.

If you do activity that suddenly alters direction, e.g. sports involving running, kicking or lifting, then it is even more important to thoroughly warm up and stretch so that you don't risk injury.

STRENGTHENING

When did you last do a handstand? Could you do one today or does the thought make you laugh? Women tend to have less and less strength unless they work or play at it. As we age we lose a certain amount of muscle strength. Injury, inactivity and all the time-saving devices can reduce the muscular fitness needed to keep our bodies strong.

Strengthening is naturally achieved when you do any activity over time. Walking, swimming, biking, and tennis are examples where you are benefiting your heart as well as strengthening your body. However, overdoing and overusing some strengthening exercises, such as hitting with a racket one-handed, long periods of cycling or twisting one way to hit a ball, can lead to injury, imbalances and pain.

The strengthening exercises in the posture workout are done in a hold position (e.g. maintaining a squat), or moving (e.g. lifting a weight up and down). Both approaches can be made more or less vigorous – you can vary the length of holding and change the weight of what you move up and down. This will counteract repetitive movements you may not realize you are doing every day.

Do a combination of strengthening exercises where you both hold and move your body.

Hold: try to hold for about 10 seconds.

Move: do sets of 3 to 6, resting between each set for about 20 seconds.

30 minutes of moderate physical activity on most days, with some huffing and puffing on at least 3 of them, is extremely important for general strengthening and cardiovascular fitness.

The posture workout is a script you can modify to meet your own needs. If an area of your body is causing concern, such as a neck problem, read Chapter 8, page 115, so you can utilize specific recommendations to make the basic posture workout personal for you.

Note: The following postures and exercises are not intended to replace treatment or advice for injury. It is always advisable to get a health professional to check out your body before commencing any exercise, fitness or change of lifestyle program. I recommend you seek advice from your doctor, physiotherapist or other health professional.

If you have any of the symptoms listed below, then you need a check-up from your doctor:

- *Unexplained weight loss*

- *Unexplained pain at night*

- *Unexplained bleeding from anywhere*

- *Feel generally unwell*

- *Experience severe pain down legs / leg weakness*

- *Loss of bladder or bowel control*

BASIC POSTURES

STANDING

To achieve a beautiful, upright posture, you need to lengthen and pull yourself up through your torso.

- *Elongate the curves of spine by tucking in tummy muscles.*

- *Glide neck and chin in without tilting or tipping head, so eyes remain level.*

- *Let shoulders fall back and down in a relaxed manner.*

- *Without pushing breasts out or moving shoulders or chest, keep weight evenly balanced up through both legs.*

- *Stand evenly on arches of feet, so your weight is distributed through the pads of all toes and the heels.*

- *Your body alignment should be straight down a plumb line, so that seen from the side, your ears, shoulders, hips and knees are all in line.*

- *Reflect your vision.*

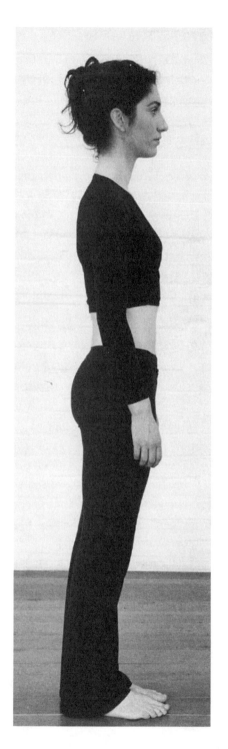

WALKING

- Hold torso erect by pulling in tummy muscles. Breathe gently and deeply.

- Ears should be in line with shoulders, and keep eyes and head level.

- Lift head and neck up from shoulders as you move.

- Incline plumb line just slightly forward to assist in propelling your body (the further forward the faster you go).

- Drive body by pumping arms to the front of chest.

- Take even strides using a heel/toe action. Think about having fluidity of movement, i.e. think of walking as a graceful, Zen-like movement.

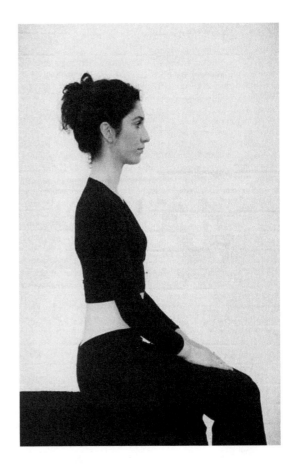

SITTING

Working

- Keep head level (imagine a glass of water balanced on your head).

- Do not tip head down to look at work for longer than a 20-minute period before bringing eyes back to level for a 5-minute break.

- Maintain spinal curve in back with support where possible.

- Sit on butt bones, butt far back in seat.

- Keep thighs level, feet flat on floor, knees at right angles.

- If you need to lean forward, move from hips, not at bra level, keeping plumb line straight.

- Do not write for longer than 20 minutes without taking a few minutes' break.

- Do not hold phone with chin and shoulder unless you change your position often.

- Get out of habit of looking over to side of computer (ideally pages you are working from should be between monitor and keyboard).

- From side-on view, ears should be in line with shoulders.

- *Maintain neck and try a change of seating, e.g. turn chair around and sit reversed, sit on floor with legs crossed, sit with pillow or support behind back.*

- *Use good lighting to read or relax with.*

- *Do not fall asleep in chair.*

LYING

ON SIDE

- *Have one-and-a-half pillows under neck, the half pillow being a soft, moldable, punch-into-shape one that stays there, so you can curl it into the gap at base of neck as support.*

- *Tuck a pillow underneath top leg to stop spine from twisting or rotating (this may stop a rolling together if you have a sleeping partner, or if you find you are uncomfortable when you waken).*

ON BACK

- *You should require only one smaller pillow.*

- *Try another pillow under knees to relax low back curve.*

- *Check that sleeping surface suits you.*

ON TUMMY

- *Have one knee bent up, one leg straight out, head turned to one side. In this position the spine is actually relaxed and in a fairly neutral shape.*

Note: *You should be careful of this position if you have a neck problem.*

POSTURE WORKOUT

The following three exercises can be described as the top three exercises for good posture. Use these as a posture quick-fix and also as a warm-up before beginning the full posture workout, which starts with the neck exercises.

1)   BREATHING

- *Smooth out face and calm mind.*
- *Close eyes (optional).*
- *Open chest position by pulling shoulders back and down, and let shoulders remain relaxed and down as you breathe.*
- *Keep mouth relaxed, try to breathe in (inhale) through nose, then let yourself breathe out (exhale) through mouth.*
- *Breathe in slowly over 5 counts, then breathe out over the same count for 5.*
- *Do 3 to 5 breaths in one set, take a moment, then do another set.*
- *Perform this type of breathing throughout the day.*

You can do this breathing exercise adding a tummy muscle contraction (exercise 2) or pelvic tilt (page 123).

2)   ABDOMINAL BRACING (TUMMY BRACE)

Using the tummy brace daily will help to keep your abdominal muscles toned.

Note: To prevent back problems, always tummy brace as you lift or when you push or pull. Use the brace action if you are sitting for over an hour at a time, or stationary such as during a long car ride. This will help to support your spine and take away stiffness.

To feel how to brace, place hands on either side of waist, fingers on tummy, and give a good cough – try to feel the tensioning of your abdominal wall.

- *Without the cough, do the tummy brace.*
- *Breathe as you brace and build up your ability to do this same action easily, in any position.*
- *Try to be able to hold it for up to 10 seconds comfortably.*
- *Repeat two or three times, as often during the day as you wish.*

3)   PELVIC FLOOR CONTRACTIONS

Exercise the pelvic floor muscles *after* emptying the bladder, not during emptying (stopping the flow is just a test to ensure the correct movement – see page 36).

FIRST ACTION

- *Do a rapid, isolated squeeze or clamping action of the openings of vagina, bladder (urethra) and bowel (anus).*

- *Do these rapid, strong flick actions at about one per second.*

- Do not *hold your breath as you do them, or tighten other muscles (buttock, inner thighs), or hold in tummy. You may feel tummy muscles tighten when you contract pelvic floor muscles, which is okay providing you do not make that the main sensation.*

- *Do about 4 to 6 per set and try to do two to three sets at a time, relaxing between each set since they are tiring when you do them correctly. (See* Note *below.)*

Progress from lying or sitting to focusing on good, strong contractions while standing, walking, running, lifting, coughing.

The easiest position to start in is forward lean (sitting with elbows on knees, legs apart). Sometimes sitting on a hard chair will help – feel the lift of your muscles off the chair. Lying down to exercise the pelvic floor is recommended initially if the muscles are very weak or if you know you have a prolapse of your internal organs (check with your doctor or nurse to clarify this).

Some women isolate the movement of the vagina / bladder from the anal muscles and will feel both movements independently. Either way is fine. If you are having problems with bowel leakage, you may need to concentrate on the anal muscles and achieve a good squeeze or clamp action of this sphincter in isolation.

SECOND ACTION

- *Do a longer, more intense contraction where you try to squeeze and lift your pelvic floor muscles up inside.*

- *Squeeze and lift inside while continuing to breathe. Try to imagine the internal walls of the vagina withdrawing inside as you lift.*

- *Try for three 10-second holds that you can increase to up to ten 10-second holds.*

- *Rest for 20 seconds in between each hold.*

Note: When trying to tone up your pelvic floor muscles it is recommended that you do an initial, intensive, six-week program of pelvic floor exercises, doing 2 or 3 sets up to 6 times a day. This six-week intensive start will really improve your muscles, and with regular exercise they will continue to support you over life. Research has shown that a better overall improvement of the strength and co-ordination of the muscles comes from a blend of the two actions described above.

NECK

Exercises 4 and 5 will keep your neck supple and allow you to hold your head and neck in a beautiful posture.

4)   NECK GLIDING

- *Sit with straight back, head level, feet flat on floor.*

- *Tuck in chin so head moves slightly backwards, without any tilting or tipping.*

- *Repeat this movement slowly (up to 10 times) so you feel your neck glide smoothly. This will loosen all your neck joints. It should feel as if you are reversing a poking-chin posture.*

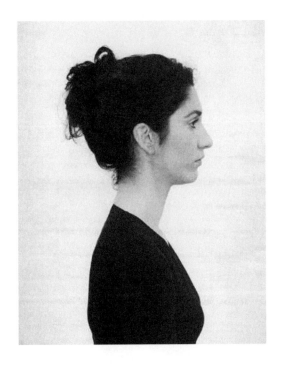 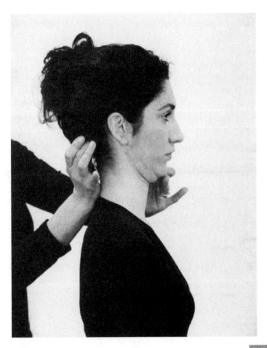

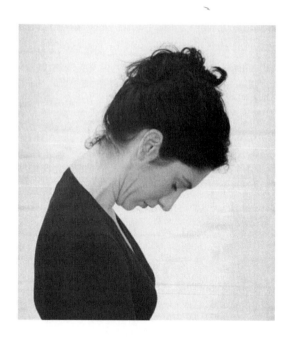

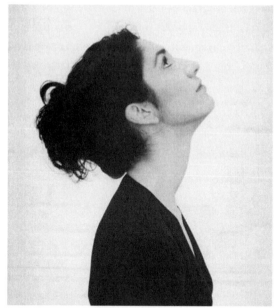

5)   NECK STRETCH UP AND DOWN

- Sit with straight back, head level, feet flat on floor.

- Keeping mouth closed, try to first put chin onto chest, stretching back of neck, then look upwards to ceiling and stretch front of neck.

- Do this slowly, about 5 times, and feel the stretch through muscles up and down neck and even in upper back.

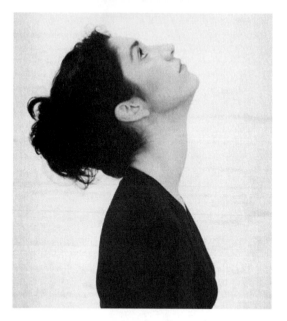

Exercises 6 and 7 will strengthen your neck safely and are very good if your neck is sore or weak from a previous injury. With these two exercises you do not need to move your neck, just tense up the muscles.

6) NECK STRENGTHENING, SIDE TO SIDE

- *Place palm of hand on side of face, push with head and neck and resist this movement with hand. Feel the tension up through the neck muscles on that side.*

- *Hold for count of 5, then slowly release.*

- *Repeat three times.*

- *Repeat on other side.*

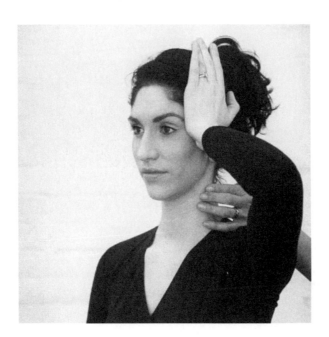

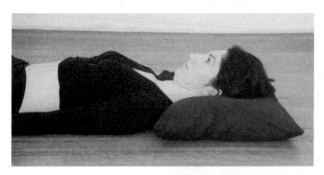

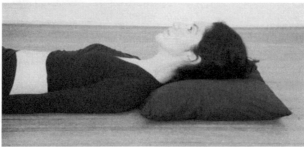

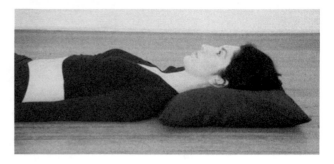

7) NECK STRENGTHENING, FRONT TO BACK

You may find it easier to lie down to do both parts of this exercise.

- *Lift head just off pillow, then press head against pillow.*

- *Place hands on forehead, press head against hands. You will feel this in muscles on either side of front of neck.*

- *Then place hands behind head and press back against them. You will feel this at base of head.*

- *Hold each tensioning for count of 5, then slowly release.*

- *Repeat the two positions 3 times.*

CHEST AND UPPER BACK

The goal of exercises 8–11 is to allow you to hold your shoulders and chest in a correct position without effort or strain.

8)   CHEST STRETCHES

Choose a position that allows you to comfortably stretch your chest and shoulder muscles. The seated stretch (B) is a good exercise at a workstation when you need to take a break. The standing stretch (C) is excellent if you have to stand for long periods.

A) LYING CHEST STRETCH

- *Lie on back with knees bent and pelvis tilted upwards so spine is flat on floor. Use a pillow to support head if you wish.*

- *Place hands behind neck, then pull elbows back gradually, aiming to rest them on floor. You will feel this stretch in your chest.*

- *Keep spine flat, keep breathing gently.*

- *Hold for 30 seconds.*

- *Repeat three times, stretching a little further each time.*

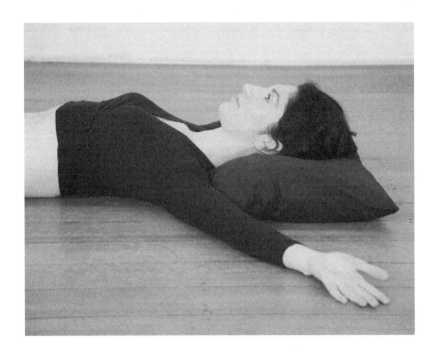

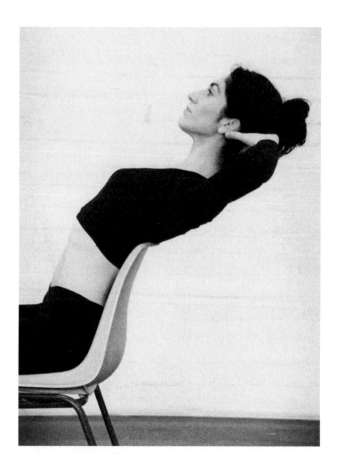

B) SEATED CHEST STRETCH

- *Sit with feet flat on floor, shift butt to back of chair as far as possible, so that chair is supporting spine.*

- *Place hands behind head, then arch back over back of chair and pull elbows back to stretch out upper chest and shoulder region.*

- *Hold for about 30 seconds.*

- *Keep head and neck relaxed, keep breathing and look up gently and slowly.*

C) STANDING CHEST STRETCH

- *Stand in a doorway, lift elbows to shoulder height and rest forearms and palms against sides of door frame.*

- *Place one leg out in front of the other so you are in a step position. This allows you to control this movement well, and as you step through the doorway, you will feel the stretch through chest and shoulders.*

- *Hold for 30 seconds, then slowly release.*

- *Repeat 3 times.*

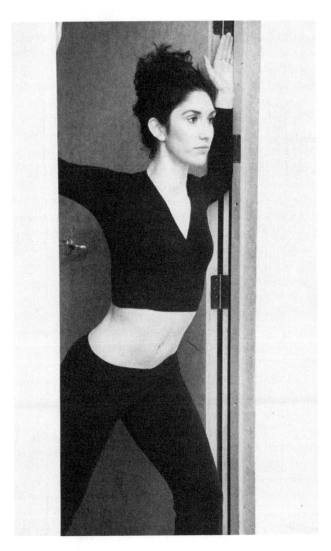

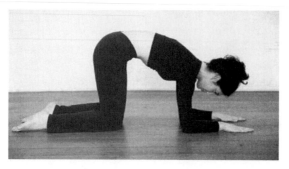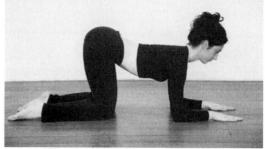

9)   ARCH OF THE CAT

This stretches your entire spine. It is a "down on hands and knees," yoga-style stretch. A combination of (A) and (B) is great for spinal mobility.

A) FOR MID AND UPPER BACK

- *Begin on forearms and knees.*
- *Pull tummy in, look down to floor.*
- *Slowly round back, arching it up.*
- *Reverse this to gently hollow back.*
- *Repeat up to 10 times as you continue to breathe in a relaxed manner.*

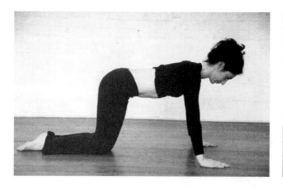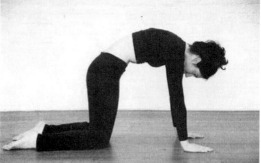

B) FOR LOWER BACK

- *Start on hands and knees.*
- *Do the movements in (A) above.*

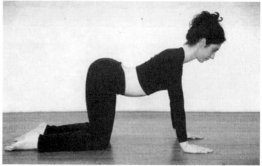

10) CHEST STRENGTHENING

While it is recommended that you keep your upper trunk flexible for good posture, this group of muscles also needs to be strong to support your spine all day. Choose an exercise from the following that you can do easily, then challenge yourself with a more difficult progression.

Note: Many women today do not keep their upper body (arms, chest and upper back) fit – by this I mean work out in a physical manner such as lifting, racquet sports, gardening or housework. If this is you, then combinations of exercises 10 and 11 will help you to maintain good muscle tone and therefore help achieve good posture.

A) STATIC CHEST STRENGTHENING

- *Put hands in front of chest as if praying.*
- *Press hands together so you tense chest muscles.*

- *Hold for about 10 counts.*
- *Repeat 3 to 5 times.*

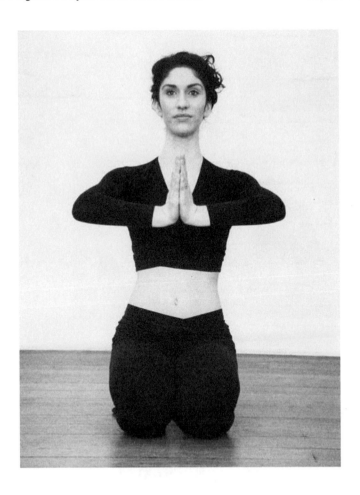

B) *Bench press*

- *Lie on back holding a weight in each hand above shoulders with arms straight.*

- *Lower weights to chest, allowing elbows to point outwards.*

- *Push weights up directly above shoulders, 6 to 8 times.*

- *Do 3 sets.*

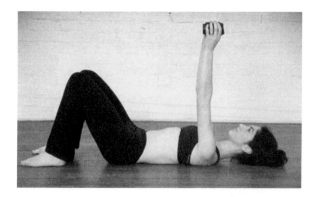

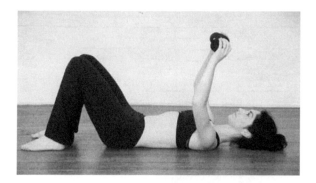

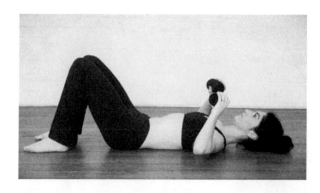

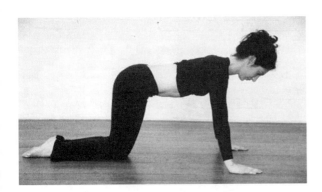

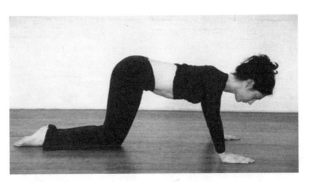

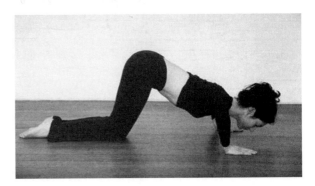

C) HALF PUSH-UPS

- *Begin on hands and knees.*

- *Breathe in, and by taking elbows out to side, lower chest to ground.*

- *Breathe out and push chest back up.*

- *Keep body straight throughout this movement by pulling tummy in firmly.*

- *Repeat 10 times.*

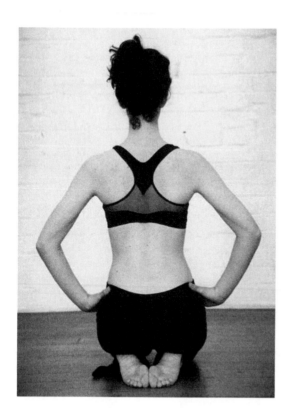 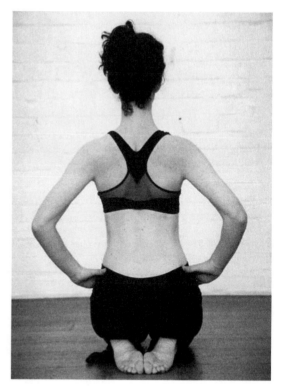

11)   UPPER BACK STRENGTHENING

- *In a sitting, standing or lying position, rest hands on hips and squeeze shoulder blades together.*

- *Hold for 10 seconds, then release.*

- *Repeat 5 to 10 times, do often through the day.*

PROGRESSIONS

A) PRONE SHOULDER STRENGTHENING

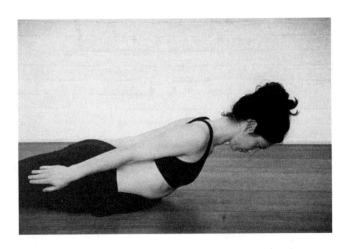

- Lie on tummy, with pillow under hips.

- While squeezing shoulder blades together, look downwards and lift shoulders off floor.

- Try to hold lift for about 20 seconds.

- Repeat 10 times.

B) BENT-OVER ROWING

- Stand, or sit on edge of seat with knees slightly bent.

- Keep back flat and lean forward from hips.

- With straight arms, hold weights just in front of knees and pull weights toward chest as if rowing.

- Repeat 6 to 8 times for 3 sets.

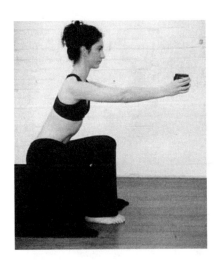
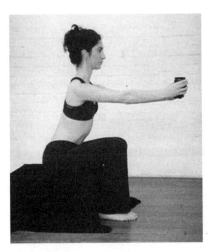
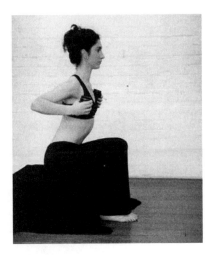

SHOULDERS

While it is not necessary to do shoulder exercises to maintain good posture, if your shoulders catch or are achy when you move, it is useful to have a range of exercises to keep them supple. You can do a selection of these regularly, preferably each day to ensure your shoulders are kept in good condition.

12)   PENDULAR EXERCISES

- *Lean forward as if going to bowl a ball, with one arm on your other knee or resting on a table.*

- *Do following movements with other arm, 10 times each:*
  - *swing forwards and backwards*
  - *circle both ways, clockwise and counter-clockwise*
  - *swing across and out away from body*

- *Turn around and repeat with other arm.*

- *Repeat for a total of about 5 minutes to loosen up shoulders.*

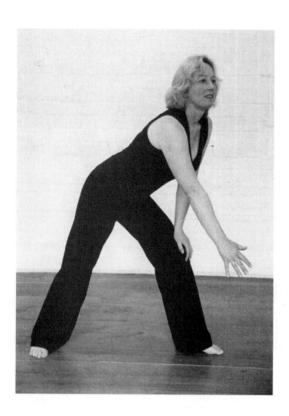 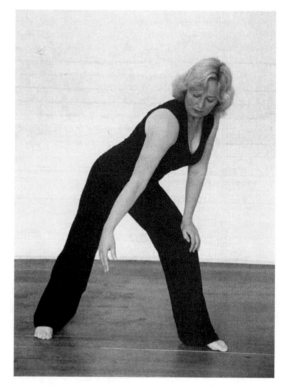

13) TOWEL DRYING

To improve reaching behind back:

- *After a bath or shower put towel around back and dry back and butt with towel in hands.*

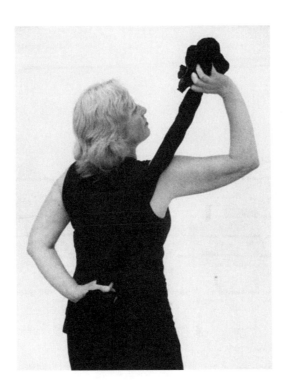

14) SKULLING IN WATER

To help sore and stiff shoulders:

- *In a deep bath, spa or pool, let arms float away from body.*
- *Keeping fingers together so hands act as paddles, do figure eights in water, using the water as a resistance to slowly and safely stretch and strengthen arms.*

15)   ASSISTED SHOULDER LIFT

- *With a hand at each end, hold an umbrella or golf club horizontally in front of body, just away from tummy.*

- *From one end, push the other end out to side, working arms like the pendulum on a clock.*

- *Increase the lift as shoulders warm up and loosen.*

- *Repeat for a minute.*

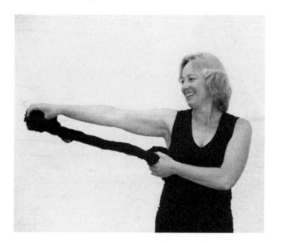 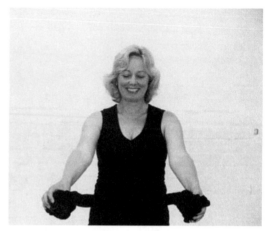

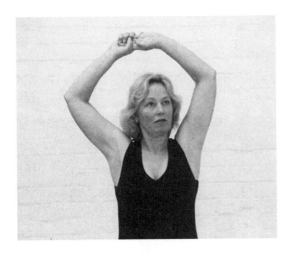 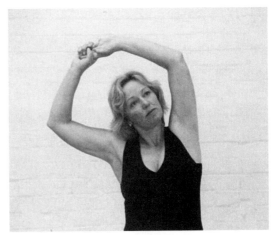

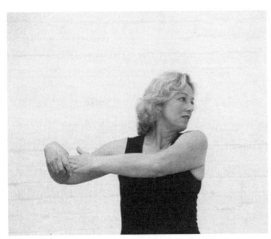 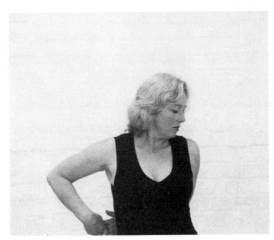

16)   ROTATOR CUFF THREE-WAY STRETCH

This stretches all the main muscles around your shoulder.

- *Hold one hand with the other and lift it:*
  - *- up and over head*
  - *- then across in front of body*
  - *- then behind back*

  Feel the stretch in shoulder joint.

- *Hold each position for the count of 5.*

- *Repeat with other arm, 3 times each arm.*

17) POLISH THE TABLE

- *The simple task of polishing a table, using circular, forward and backward movements, will strengthen the shoulders.*

18) PUSH-UPS

This is a full push-up, a progression of exercise 10C, page 87.

- *Begin on hands and knees, hands a shoulder-width apart and feet almost together.*

- *Incline body forward slightly so you can lift knees off ground. Your body will now be supported in a straight line with hands in front of feet.*

- *Breathe in and lower body to ground by bending elbows, aiming to nearly touch chest to ground.*

- *Breathe out and push body back to raised position.*

- *Widen the distance between hands to increase the arm and shoulder strengthening effect.*

- *Repeat 6 to 8 times.*

Note: This exercise is difficult and requires caution if you have shoulder problems.

19) COMBO SHOULDER LIFT

This simple exercise is a combination of two exercises, so saves you time.

- *Take a weight in each hand, 1 to 2 lbs.*

- *Start with arms by sides.*

- *Keeping arms straight, but not locking elbows, lift weights to shoulder height along a diagonal (in a direction halfway between forward and sideways), and lower them again.*

- *Make sure you keep elbows ever-so-slightly bent so that you do not strain them.*

- *Do 3 sets of 6 to 8.*

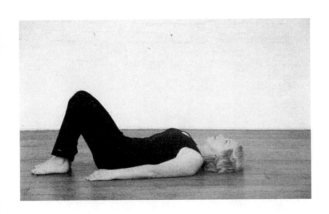 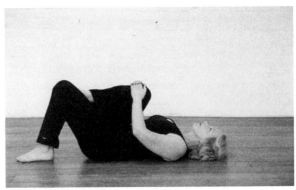

LOWER BACK

20)   STRETCH INTO FLEXION (PULL KNEES TO CHEST)

- *Lie on back with knees bent.*
- *Use hands to bring knees alternately onto chest, hold for a count of 5, then release.*
- *Do three 3 on each leg.*

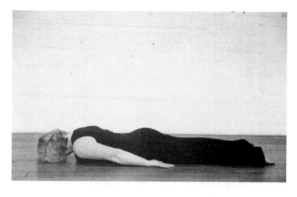 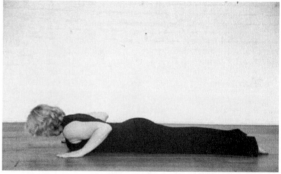

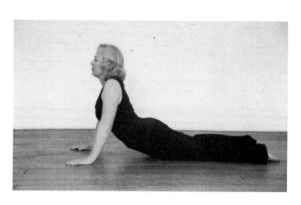

21) STRETCH INTO EXTENSION
(ARCH UP)

- *Lie on tummy, place arms so that hands are in line with shoulders.*

- *Press upper body off floor, keep buttocks relaxed and go up until you feel hips start to come off surface.*

- *Breathe out, then slowly lower.*

- *Repeat up to 10 times.*

22) BALANCE

Balancing is a very good way to strengthen your whole body. You are working really hard by doing this and it is also fun.

- *Begin on hands and knees.*

- *Lift an opposite arm and leg straight up off the floor.*

- *Hold trunk still and firm for about 30 seconds.*

- *Repeat 3 times.*

Try it lying flat on tummy and then progress to lying with your body lengthways over a narrow beam – a line of cushions or a foam block will suffice.

ABDOMINALS AND BUTTOCKS

A balance between these two muscle groups will give you a nice shape and a nice feel. To work this area effectively, I believe a combination of stretching and strengthening, including basic cardiovascular fitness is the way to go. Get into the habit of consistently doing the static abdominal brace (exercise 2, page 75).

23)   BEST-EVER ABDOMINAL EXERCISE PROGRAM

A) UP, UP, DOWN, DOWN

This is a great way to safely exercise your lower and deep abdominal muscles.

- *Lie on back with knees bent.*

- *Flatten back down against the surface you are on and brace tummy.*

- *Lift one knee to 90 degrees, then the other; lower one leg, then lower the other to go back to starting position. Repeat as often as you like – 20 is a good number.*

- *Remember to breathe out as you clench your abdominals.*

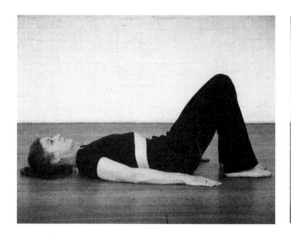
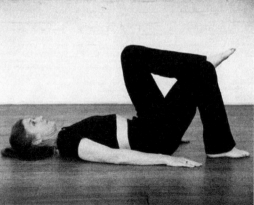
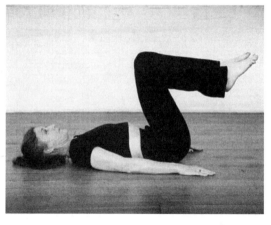
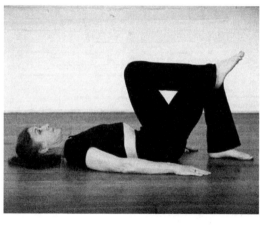

B) *Single leg slides*

- *Begin as in (A) above.*

- *Brace and lift one knee to 90 degrees, then stretch other leg so you slide it out straight along floor, then return to starting position.*

- *Repeat with other leg.*

- *By keeping your sliding leg off the floor, it adds more leverage to the spine, so be careful if you have a sore low back.*

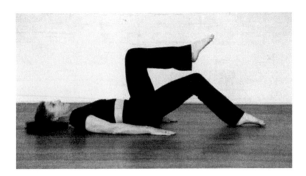

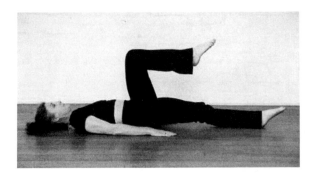

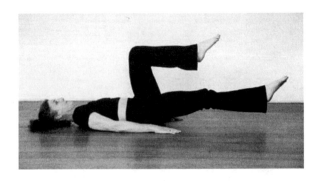

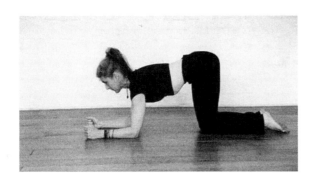

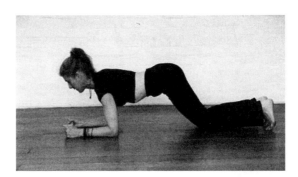

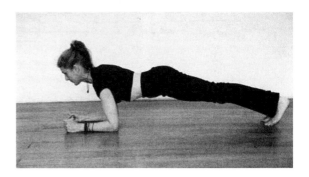

C) *STATIC ABDOMINAL HOLD*

- *Begin on forearms and knees.*

- *Keeping forearms and feet on floor, lift knees off floor.*

- *Hold for 10–20 seconds. As you support your body, keeping it as firm as you can, your entire trunk gets a workout – awesome for the whole body, and very difficult.*

- *Repeat 3 times.*

D) OBLIQUE ABDOMINALS

- *Lie on back, lift legs so heels are directly above hips.*

- *With knees slightly bent, lower legs over to one side slowly until you feel opposite shoulder wants to lift off floor.*

- *Use abdominal muscles on the sides to pull legs back to upright.*

- *Repeat 6 to 8 times each way.*

- *Keep tummy braced as you do this exercise.*

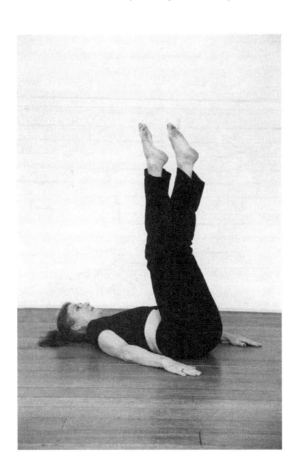 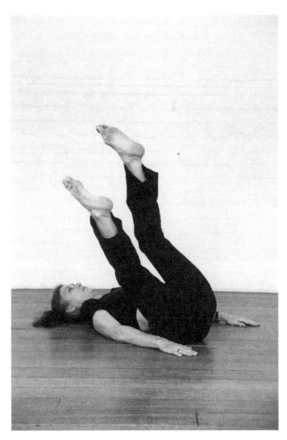

Buttocks and hips

24) Butt stretch

This is a stretch to target your buttock. You should feel an ache right in the cheek.

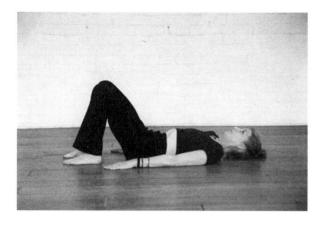

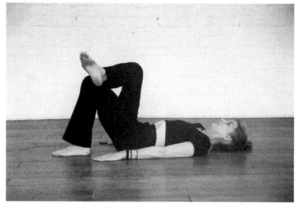

A) PIRIFORMIS MUSCLE STRETCH IN LYING

- *Lie on back with knees bent.*
- *Place right ankle onto left knee.*
- *Take hold of left thigh and pull leg towards chest – you will feel a stretch in the right buttock.*
- *Hold for 20–30 seconds, then release slowly and gently.*
- *Repeat 3 times with each leg.*

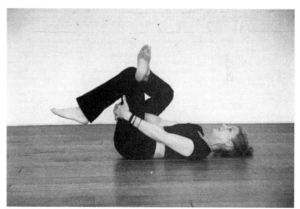

B) PIRIFORMIS MUSCLE STRETCH IN STANDING

- *Stand with one foot on a chair seat or low stool.*

- *Let the leg on chair slowly push back, then stretch body forward from hips, hand reaching down this leg.*

- *Slightly bend knee of standing leg.*

- *Feel a stretch in buttock that is pushed back.*

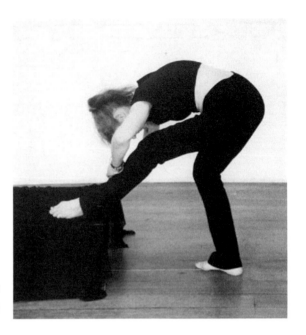

25)   BUTT STRENGTHENING

All these strengthening exercises work the legs as well as the buttocks and improve your general fitness.

B) STEP-UPS

- *Step up and down with alternate legs, just as you would to climb stairs.*

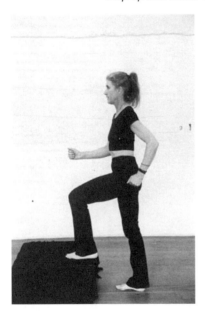
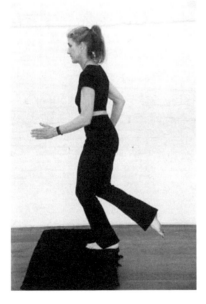

C) STEP-DOWNS (VARIATION)

- *Facing down a step, stand with one leg on the step, the other off to the side or off the edge of the step.*

- *Step down so that the toes of one leg just touch the ground lightly, then drive back up with that leg.*

- *Repeat 5 times, then change legs.*

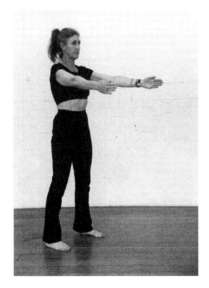 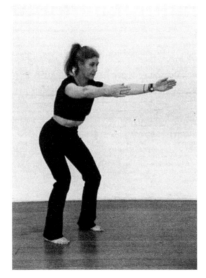 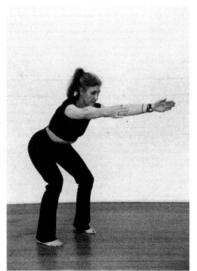

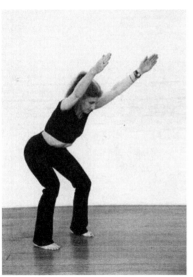 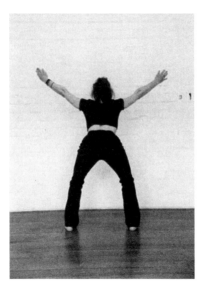

D) HALF SQUATS

This is a natural strengthening exercise because you are using your own body weight, and to do it properly requires you to keep your torso nice and firm.

Note: Be careful with this exercise if you have painful, weak or stiff legs.

- *Stand with heels on ground, legs shoulder-width apart.*

- *Lean forward from hips and sink into a squat, bending knees to slightly less than 90 degrees.*

- *Keep looking straight ahead.*

- *Drive back up using butt and tummy muscles.*

- *Do about 20 at a time.*

LEGS

A great workout for your legs includes any weight-bearing activity such as walking, mowing lawns, gardening, cycling, jogging, aerobics. Where the emphasis is on improving your posture try to have a variety of these activities during your week.

Stretching your legs will help to strengthen them more effectively. Both stretching and strengthening increases circulation and helps to counteract problems like aching legs from standing all day.

Note: For exercises 26–28 stretch one leg for a 20-second hold, slowly release, then do on other leg. Repeat 3 times.

26) FRONT OF THIGH STRETCH

A) SIMPLE HIP FLEXOR STRETCH

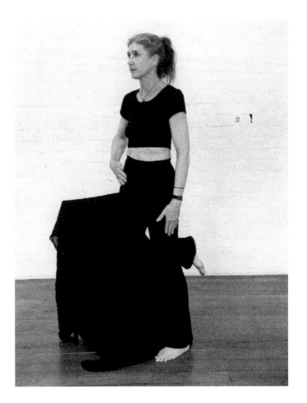

- *Stand and pull in tummy muscles.*

- *Place one knee on a chair so shin is resting on seat of chair.*

- *Push hip forward on that side so you are placing a gentle stretch on front of hip.*

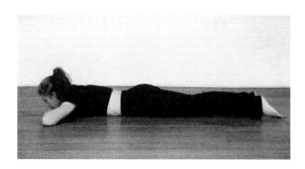

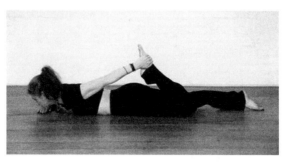

B) *ALTERNATIVE HIP FLEXOR STRETCH*

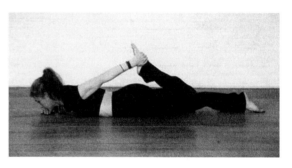

- *Lie on tummy or side, bend up one leg behind you and take hold of ankle.*

- *Pull in tummy muscles.*

- *Stretch front of thigh by pushing this hip forward.*

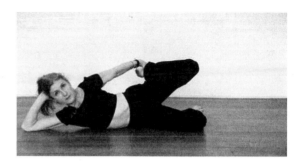

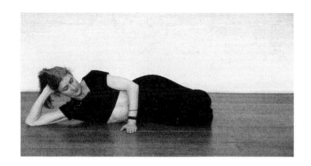

C) LUNGE

Note: This exercise needs caution if you have a knee problem.

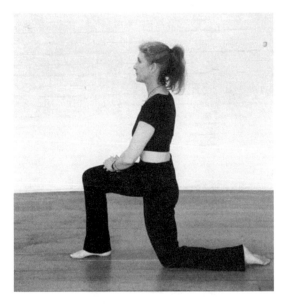

- *Kneel so you are in a lunge, with front foot flat on floor, knee at 90-degree angle, and back shin resting on floor.*

- *Place both hands on front knee for balance.*

- *Lean forward at hips so back leg is stretching up through front of hip and thigh.*

- *Do not arch back too much.*

- *Keep hips facing forward.*

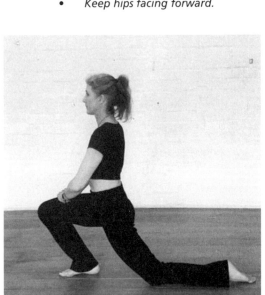

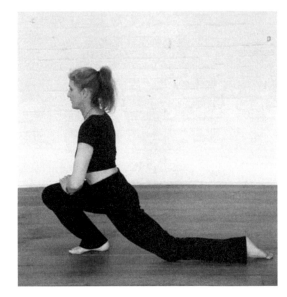

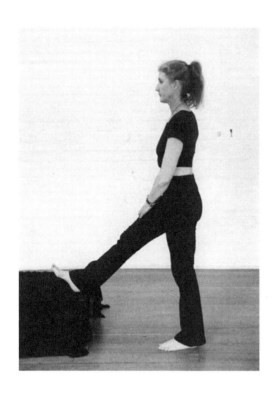

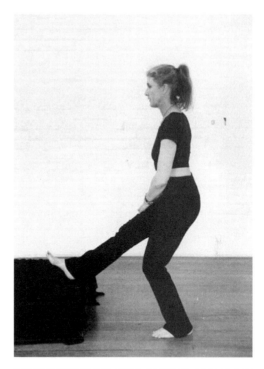

27) BACK OF THIGH STRETCH

A) HAMSTRING STRETCH IN STANDING

- *Place one leg on a chair or low table.*

- *Keep balance with both hands on front leg.*

- *Bend leg you are standing on slightly and lean body forward to stretch up back of leg.*

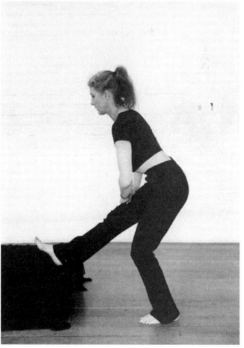

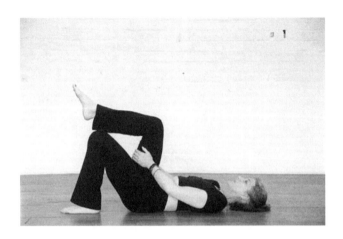

B) HAMSTRING STRETCH IN LYING

- Lie on floor with one knee bent.

- Stretch other leg into air, supporting leg with hands.

- Try for a 90-degree angle with a relatively straight leg.

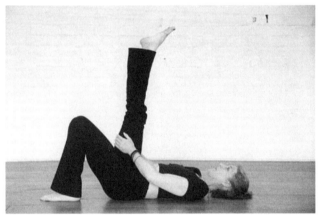

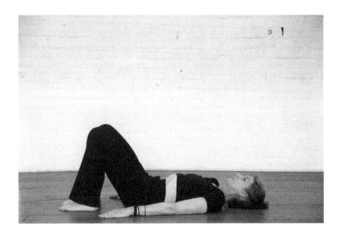

28) CALF MUSCLE STRETCH

- *Stand with one foot a step in front of the other.*

- *Bend front leg, and keeping heels down, lean forward until you feel a gentle stretch up back of calf muscle.*

- *Then bend back leg and stretch a little further.*

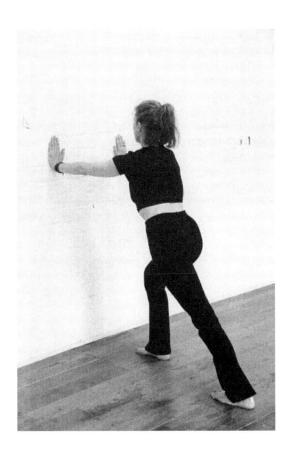 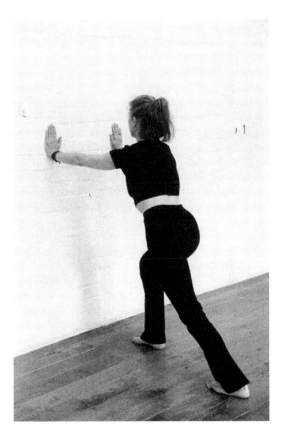

29) LEG STRENGTHENING AND BALANCING

A good test for leg strength is to be able to stand for 30 seconds on each leg with no wobbling or tipping of your pelvis. Any weakness in your legs will often show up when you try this – if it is easy, try it with your eyes closed and test your balance without your visual receptors (eyes). You have to rely on your legs to give you the correct positional information.

- *Any aerobic activity will enhance the strength in your legs. Weight-bearing activities such as walking are especially good for maintaining bone density.*

MICROMOVES

Micromoves, or good posture on the go, are designed to enhance your body awareness and release the stress and tension that collects in certain areas, blocking nutrition and blood flow and causing pain. We are not talking sweat pants and leotards – more about simply taking a deep breath, wiggling your toes, or stretching your shoulders and upper back. These micromoves are like a postural yawn or blink, to allow you to refocus.

You can create many opportunities in your day to use these cute little movements to stimulate your body, refresh your mind and energize your soul. That supermarket line is the perfect place to put the power of posture into action, to develop body awareness and feel how the ideal alignment of your body tones up your system. So what could you do in the supermarket? Exercises 1–3 in the posture workout are all perfect.

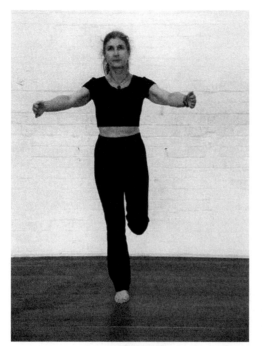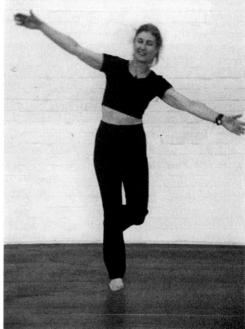

If you are becoming very static in your daily tasks while coping with an ever-growing workload, your body will feel as if it is beginning to get rusty. So use the micromoves, do the split-second, tiny, effortless actions to keep your body (your machine) purring like a kitten. Take a moment whenever possible to keep as loose as a goose and supple as a cat, toned to the max!

WAYS TO MICROMOVE

Use exercises 1–3 in the workout as your ultimate micromoves.

Do these in any position you wish

Nodding, tilting or turning your head just 10 degrees (your skull on the top neck bones) gives you tiny movements to keep your neck supple.

Lift neck off shoulders by making yourself tall.

Close eyes for a moment.

Yawn.

Stretch body after your yawn.

Shrug and pull shoulders down.

Move shoulders alternately forwards / middle / backwards.

Stretch arms as long as possible.

Swing arms loosely, conducting an imaginary orchestra.

Circle wrists.

Stretch fingers as long as possible.

Clench and release fingers.

Play drums with fingers.

March on the spot either in standing or sitting.

Buttock clenches in sitting / standing / lying.

In standing

Stand on one leg, stopping hip from dropping.

Stand on one leg, keep your balance with eyes closed.

Rise up and down on toes.

Stretch body forward, bend knees and roll body down to touch ground with hands.

In sitting

Reach arms up to the ceiling.

Kick out alternate legs to straighten knees, and hold.

Squeeze knees together, count for 5.

Foot and ankle circles.

Dig heels into floor.

Press your back into the chair.

Push head back against the headrest.

The lower torso section (tummy) and pelvic floor platform (underneath and de...

hold the key - in a postural sense - to our bodies, but also throughout time it h...

Influencing and directing the changes that happen to this es...

...inside us) make up the unique part of a woman. Not only does this part of us ...een associated with a woman's physical, emotional and even spiritual energy. ...ial part will help you to feel the power of posture.

More energy

Define who YOU are

Enhance your sexuality

Develop physical power

Positive aging

— get older and better!

HEADACHES

I believe most simple headaches come from poor neck posture and the tension we carry there. Headaches and achy shoulders are often simply a result of a postural droop. People have told me that in the morning, driving to work, they look out the top section of the windshield, but when they drive home at the end of the day they find they are looking through a lower part of the windshield because they have curved their back over from sitting all day, and have become tired. But they tell me they don't do this on vacation, even though they do a lot of driving – probably because they are having a regular change of position, usually including a walking activity, and are less stressed.

To relieve the tension across the neck and back of shoulders which so often leads to a headache, do exercises 4, 5, 7, 8, 10 and 16 in the posture workout daily.

Avoiding headaches

Do the "steps to relaxation" (see page 55) and focus on feeling heavy and warm especially around your head, neck and upper shoulders.

Take regular breaks about every 20 minutes. Use natural breaks in your tasks, or divide work into sections and take a break after completing each little section.

Do micromoves:
- *Squeeze and release the muscles around shoulders and neck, to stimulate relaxation*
- *Hunch the shoulders and let go*
- *Pull shoulder blades together, then let go*
- *Stretch arms out, then let go*
- *Open fingers and hands, stretch, then let go*
- *Use your breathing to take a moment*
- *Make sure you keep hydrated with fluid*

NECK

Beautiful, relaxed neck posture comes from the muscles not having to work hard to hold you upright. Your head is balanced comfortably on your shoulders. Picture yourself with an upright, curved but elegant neck that is held firmly. Muscles in the front, deep in your throat, and at the sides and back of your neck all play a part in keeping you supported. Viewed from the side, your ears should be level with your shoulders at all times. If your ears go forward of this neutral position, as when your head and eyes drop down to read, not only does this become your habitual position to read in, but it puts stress and tension on your neck muscles. Combining exercises 4 and 5 in the workout stretches the tiny joints and muscles at the base of the skull and will often make a headache vanish.

> *Glide your neck in (see page 77), then tip chin down to chest, come back to level and repeat the neck glide as you look up to ceiling.*

If your neck is giving you problems, you should look at your whole body and try to see if there is anything in your posture that has altered lately. Many people place their head off to one side as a matter of habit, especially with answering phones or just from being left- or right-handed, and simply addressing this can help to successfully manage a neck problem. This means thinking about how you talk on the phone. Think about the work you are doing, and whether it is maybe off to one side of the keyboard for instance. Be wary if you spend time in static postures such as at a sewing machine. It is quite scary to think how static even children's bodies are becoming, and the increasing pace of lifestyles consumes us all.

The joints in the neck are delicate and complex. Car accidents and whiplashes from sports and other accidents can trouble people for years. Getting a tune-up from a health professional can clear these joints, unblock the movements and correct some mechanical faults.

DOWAGER'S HUMP

If you place both hands up around your neck, fingers pointing to your back, they join at the base of the neck and the beginning of the spine – the junction of the cervical vertebrae in your neck and the thoracic vertebrae in your spine. Your ribs come in here as well and many muscles attach and work from this point.

A dowager's hump is a fatty pad of thickened connective tissue over the top of this area of your spine. It is ugly, painful, accentuated with poor posture and more evident in women with osteoporosis. It cannot be cut out or removed surgically.

Your posture is the key to prevention of this condition. If you are developing a lump you will need a safe and effective postural program to reverse or halt the effects of gravity, time, hard work or old age.

Note: If you have osteoporosis, you may need to be very gentle when putting yourself into positions that cause pain. It is important to keep yourself as strong as possible. Check with a physiotherapist.

I recommend regularly doing the posture workout exercises 4–7 for both dowager's hump and neck problems. Two extra exercises you may find beneficial are:

1) Slowly turn head to the side, breathing out.

Look behind you and hold for count of 5.

Repeat on other side.

2) Slowly take head sideways, ear toward shoulder, breathing out.

Do not raise shoulders or let head tip forward.

Repeat on other side.

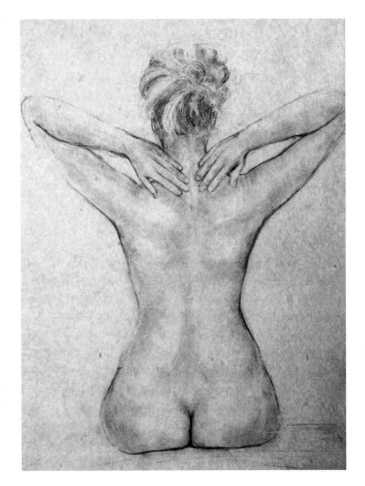

SHOULDERS

Bone densitometry will check bone thickness and quality to guage any thinning of the bones (osteoporosis). Discuss this with your doctor if you are over 50 or have the following risk factors:

- Too skinny and no body fat
- History in your family of osteoporosis
- Poor diet (deficient in calcium and vegetables) when you were young
- Loss of ovaries at an early age
- Postmenopausal
- A lifestyle that involves hunching over computer, sewing machine, or sitting activities such as driving
- Lack of regular participation throughout your life in weight-bearing exercises such as walking or other sports

When shoulders don't work well, they seem to hinder everything we do. Shoulders that clunk as you move them can be called rough shoulders. The moving tissues in the shoulders are like ropes running over pulleys and they often get frayed and rough. Occupations that require overhead work or reaching, and repetitive movement such as keyboard work, will fatigue and wear out these ropes or tendons more rapidly.

Although the round-shouldered look is often reversible, as we age this condition becomes more permanent. When I talk posture with women they tend to pull up their shoulders, hunch them backwards, hold their breath, stick their chests out, then think – oh no, my boobs stick out – so go back to a slumped posture. To improve your posture, don't move your shoulders – lift up out of your tummy or torso, lengthen your neck, but let your shoulders be relaxed and loose. Your shoulders will settle into a good posture if you control your spine. The basic posture in standing and sitting addresses the alignment of your shoulders (see pages 72–74).

In the posture workout, exercises 12–19, pages 90–94, have been designed to target stiff and sore shoulders safely. Why not take this book with you to your therapist to check that they are suitable for you.

Note: If you have a frozen shoulder or significant shoulder problems, I recommend a diagnosis, then develop a plan of management with your health professional. Check with them on the suitability of exercises.

Upper back and chest

Sometimes we need extra effort to be able to hold ourselves well and this requires flexibility of the upper back and chest. Test your flexibility as follows:

Lie on your back on a bed, your head supported with a pillow, and let your arms relax by your side.

Where are your shoulders? They should be touching the bed, or just slightly off. If your shoulders are more than 3 to 4 inches or a fist forward of neutral, this is caused by tight chest muscles or a stiff upper spine.

Reach up and out with your arms, halfway between fully above your head and out to the side. Your arms should be able to lie flat on the bed or floor, without raising your back off the bed. If you have to bend your arms or lift your back, this too means your chest or upper back is stiff and can be giving you problems with your upper torso, including neck and shoulders.

If chest and back flexibility has become a problem for you, it highlights the importance of the posture workout. Exercises 10 and 12, pages 85 and 90, will improve this flexibility and can be simply added to your day.

Spine and lower back

Sensuously curved, beautifully shaped and an exquisite piece of architecture – I am talking about your spine. I want you to develop a love affair with your spine and to enjoy your curves. Don't ruin it by straightening it all out or sagging it out of shape when you sit or rest.

A baby develops the spinal curves as it learns to move from lying to crawling, sitting, rolling and on to walking those first tottering steps. A child moves with perfect form when they pick up a toy. They can remain comfortably squatting as they play, their spine flexible and supple and not unduly influenced by the pull of imbalanced muscles. As they get older they start to sit more, and by the time they are going to school we start to see the effect of bad postural influences on the muscles acting on their spine, affecting posture and balance. They carry heavy schoolbags on one shoulder, spend hours at computers and badly designed desks. I wonder if our children are being made fully aware of their posture so they understand how to hold themselves erect and balanced.

Low back pain

While back pain is not gender specific, from my clinical experience I believe women have back pain unique to themselves. Common spinal conditions in women include osteoarthritis (wear and tear), osteoporosis (bone thinning), disk degeneration and changes to the normal shape of your spine. This can be due to injury, or sometimes you are born with it (see photo on the following page). There is no doubt that the hormonal influences working on the ligaments to soften and stretch the pelvic canal for birth have an effect on the elasticity of the spinal tissues. Monthly cycles with the influences of hormonal peaks make a lot of women feel heavier, achier and looser in their joints. Combined with the workload of women with small children there is a stressful effect on the spine often felt all over.

Getting back to pre-birth tone takes a lot more work on postural control through exercising and awareness than we might think. Just taking up tennis again or getting to the gym will not, in my opinion, restore the body to how it was before the birth.

Often back pain is triggered by tasks involved in working around the home. Think about all the bending, twisting, pushing and pulling associated with shopping, cleaning, carrying heavy objects and caring for children. Gardening and vacuuming are well known as a cause of back ache.

If your lifestyle involves a lot of sitting the tummy is placed in a relaxed state. For this to be negated, you need exercises for the tummy such as swinging a tennis racket, hula hooping or doing more of what you see kids do out in the playground. It is difficult to activate the supporting muscles around the spine if you are sitting a lot of the day, but a simple, regular change of position will often be all you need to reduce the risk of injury to your spine. One theory is that a regular change of posture stops the muscles from getting too tired and putting pressure on your joints and ligaments. So get up and walk around the room for just a minute!

It is outside the purpose and scope of this book to diagnose and/or treat low back pain. Rather, the book encourages activity and good posture to prevent episodes of back pain. If you suffer from low back pain, I recommend a medical assessment, i.e. get it diagnosed, first.

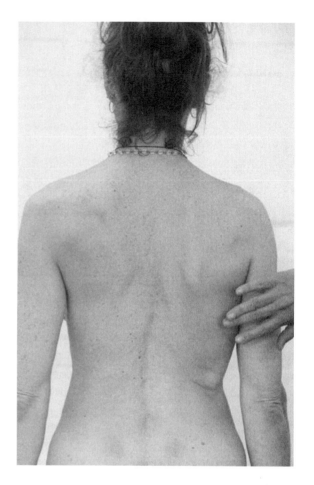

COMMON BACK SYMPTOMS

- An ache described as further up, across the bra level and into the neck and shoulders, especially when tired or after working too long in one position, such as sewing.
- Low back pain related to premenstrual times of the month, often worse mid-cycle with a sensation of a dragging-type pain in the pelvis.
- Soreness in the back from bending-over activities such as gardening or vacuuming.
- An ache in the back after sitting for over an hour, especially when the spine is unsupported such as at a sewing chair or piano stool.
- General non-specific ache from standing still for a period of time.

A sway-back posture can come from muscle imbalance between the muscles at the front and back – the tummy muscles are too long and weak and the spine muscles too short and tight. As well, the structures around the hip can be short in the front and the buttock muscles weak at the back. This can lead to an increased tendency to back pain, and is correctable with exercise programs.

Prevention of low back pain

> *Do exercises 1–3, pages 75–76, in the workout regularly through the day.*
>
> *When you come home, lie on tummy for 5 minutes.*
>
> *Lie on your back on the floor with your legs resting on the seat of a chair.*
>
> *Always arch backwards before lifting a heavy object.*

Use lumbar support in sitting.

Vary your position sitting in a chair – sit straddle, or backwards.

Sit cross-legged (like a tailor).

Garden with good postural technique.

ABDOMINALS

If you hold a balloon filled with water out in front of you, by the knot, you can see how the balloon stretches as gravity pulls it down. Imagine this as your lower torso: the sides of the balloon are your tummy and spinal muscles that wrap around your trunk, the bottom of the balloon is your pelvic floor muscles. How does your mid-section compare? Does it feel firm or a little soft and squishy?

YOUR TUMMY ...

- is a laminated, overlapping natural corset of four layers of muscle, which begins and ends at the spine.
- is like a cylinder – layers of muscle squeeze in to hold the spine firm to allow us to move effectively.
- has muscle "stays" running up the back and is sectioned across with bands in the front.
- generally has a layer of fat around the hips, which is very hormonally influenced in women.
- works better with training. This involves learning to switch the muscles on so they respond quickly as we move. For example as you hit a golf ball or throw a softball, your tummy should tighten firmly just before you connect or release.
- works best if the muscles are quick and responsive and can be a key factor in reducing episodes of low back pain.
- looks great if you do strong tummy tightening (without holding your breath!) in a variety of positions. A strong tummy is especially useful for protecting your body in lifting.

FASHION AND FAT

Through the ages the shape of the female torso has been subject to self-torment and anguish. Fashion trends have always influenced and dictated the female figure and form. For our great-grandmothers the ideal hourglass figure was achieved by being squeezed into corsets and boned in place. Some of us will remember the casual chic phase when it was very cool and groovy to slouch and display a round-shouldered, defiant-of-the-establishment sort of look. Today's models and designers often foist upon us a look that is less than elegant and certainly has nothing to do with good posture or even a healthy weight.

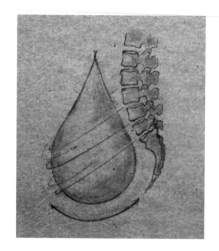

The distribution of fat over our tummies and hips (that pouch that overhangs the panty line!) is actually a good thing. This layer that rounds a woman is due partly to the hormonal effects on the body. Estrogen (the female hormone) is stored in fat cells as well as in women's ovaries and in small amounts in the adrenal glands that sit on top of the kidneys. One reason not to get too thin is so that you will not lessen your estrogen supplies for old age. Estrogen offers great protection for some of the problems that may occur in the older age group such as osteoporosis, heart disease and menopausal symptoms.

While most of us see the lower tummy as just an area where our fat seems to be, there are important reasons for making this area toned apart from controlling the sag. If you learn to control the inner and more deeply placed abdominal muscles in your lower torso this will have a big stabilizing influence on your spine – the little bones that are your spine can be braced and held steady, thus reducing the risk of low back injury. Strong lower abdominals (abs) give your pelvic floor muscles some firmness to grip against, thus supporting your internal organs and giving you a much more efficient, graceful movement when you walk. This will also often reduce hip / pelvic-type pain that women often get when they are on their feet a lot of the day. However, it is most important to do abdominal exercises correctly.

You may wish to control the fat layer with dietary modification – great. The combination of a healthy diet with toning of the muscular / skeletal system is certainly the best way to go. If you are currently on a weight-loss program, then start to think posture. As you near your ideal weight, this is the time to really tone up your body.

The dreaded crunch

Have you been one of the many who have performed countless sit-ups and crunches in order to shape up your abdominals? Feet hooked under the sofa, rolling up, straining your neck and often hurting your low back … Remember the bicycling exercise up on your elbows, backwards and forwards with the legs? Maybe you have an apparatus for your "abs" under your bed, that you get out occasionally when you feel guilty and work out on like crazy? All this encourages a posture that gives you a sort of slightly flexed, bent-over look.

Toning your tummy

You can do more for your abdominals by consciously exercising them during everyday activities. Become more aware of these muscles. When you throw a ball, the abdominal muscles should tighten and provide a stable firm trunk so you can give a nice, strong throw. If you are digging in the garden, just as you go to hit the earth with your spade the abdominal muscles should grip automatically and hold your torso so that you can safely lift up the spade plus the weight of the earth in it. Try to feel that next time you are doing these things. And go for this type of control when you are just walking.

Excellent tummy muscle exercises from the workout are exercise 2, page 75, and exercises 20–23, pages 95–97, with all progressions.

An extra exercise you may like to do is a pelvic tilt. This is a simple and lovely exercise to strengthen your tummy and mobilize your lower back gently.

Pelvic tilt

Lie on floor with knees bent.

Flatten spine onto floor, slightly tilting your pelvis. Use tummy muscles to initiate this movement.

Take pelvis further, tilting it up as much as you can.

Hold for 20–30 seconds while continuing to breathe gently.

Repeat 5–10 times.

PREGNANCY

Pregnancy changes your body in numerous ways, including subjecting the tummy muscles to being stretched and lengthened. This can weaken them and makes it harder to contract them. Don't be alarmed if you do not regain your pre-pregnancy shape right away, there is plenty of time to restore the tone. Often you will get the shape and support back with less hassle and stress when you consider your whole posture, and a woman's body can look even better when she has had a child.

Women gain on average 25 to 35 pounds during their pregnancy, but many seem to find difficulty losing this after the baby is born, and some tell me they gained considerably more than the recommended pounds. If you are pregnant or have just had a baby, use the posture workout and focus on your abdominals during activity in general. Good posture and firm tummy muscles throughout your pregnancy can be a reality but requires active muscular tone.

There is no reason not to do any of the positions and exercises outlined in this book during pregnancy. Good posture will help to support your body and avoid fatigue and aches and pains. Most women I know feel wonderfully sexual throughout their pregnancy. The whole pregnancy experience can be enhanced with vital and beautiful posture.

Note: It is especially important to strengthen the pelvic floor as you get back to physical exercise after having a baby. Try to pull up with these muscles (see exercise 3, page 76) and clench hard as you are walking along. This is quite difficult to do, but with practice you should be able to feel yourself pulling and lifting up inside to make them work even harder.

Surgery

A lot of women believe surgery accounts for lack of tone across the midriff. "After the Caesarean section, my tummy was never the same."

Post-operative instructions are usually to avoid lifting for six weeks and not overstretch the area so it heals well – but what happens? Why do women seem to lose shape and tone? Perhaps they actually lose the awareness of good support. They stop gripping the tummy as they move, and this leads to a feeling of loss of strength, and sagging develops – "if you don't use it you lose it." So after surgery it becomes very important to be aware of the tummy muscles and how to activate and use them through your day. Good posture means good firm tummy muscles.

Bladder

When your bladder gets full it sends a signal to the brain, which then talks to the pelvic floor muscles and this process gives rise to the urge to empty the bladder. The total procedure should be hassle free and without incident. However, for women in particular this does not always happen so easily.

Many of the symptoms outlined below can relate directly to poor control of the pelvic floor musculature.

Incontinence (the leakage of urine, especially with activity – "stress incontinence"). Can you sneeze, laugh or lift with a smile? Cough without crossing your legs or supporting yourself? Hit a ball without fear of a wet spot? Other forms of leakage are overflow incontinence and urge incontinence.

Urgency (the urgent need to go to the toilet). Episodes of being busting followed sometimes by leakage, especially at predictable times like first thing in the morning or arriving home.

Frequency (having to go to the toilet more often than normal). See page 125 for normal bladder habits.

Prolapse (various degrees of descent of your bladder). Other tissues that commonly prolapse are the bowel and uterus. These tissues fall into the vagina and women notice a bulge or lump, which may come and go, in their vagina. If you suspect this, recommend that your doctor confirms this condition.

Nocturia (needing to get up to pee more than once through the night). Either the urge wakes you or you are unable to sleep due to fullness in the bladder. This feeling is not just because you drink after your last meal. In fact your fluid intake and output should be roughly equal, so by the time you go to bed you have emptied out the amount of fluid you have drunk during the day and your last drink should not unduly affect your ability to sleep peacefully.

Urinary incontinence is the complaint of any involuntary leaking of urine. It is estimated that 10–25% of women under the age of 60, and 50% of women over 60 are affected by problems of prolapse and urinary incontinence.

Urinary leakage occurs with activities such as running, jumping, coughing, or with positional change such as bending down or over. It can also occur because of an inability to "hold on" until getting to the toilet. Many women believe this problem is a normal part of aging or a natural consequence of child-birth. This is not so. Pelvic floor muscle tone can be improved to give adequate bladder control at any age except sometimes where there are other complications. For instance some women may require a variety of medications, such as diuretics, or may have a lack of mobility so that getting to the toilet on time becomes too difficult.

It is interesting to note just what is considered normal bladder habits – you would be amazed at the variety of habits, which some women consider normal.

NORMAL BLADDER HABITS

- You go to the toilet on average 6 to 8 times per day.
- You do not need to get up, or get up only once, through the night to pass urine.
- You do not go for less than 2 hours or more than 4 hours without passing urine during the day.
- You pass around 10 ounces each time you empty the bladder.
- Your intake of fluid is 50 to 70 ounces of fluid per day.

Note: Always lean forward on the toilet to ensure that you empty the bladder properly.

TESTING YOUR BLADDER

This test will allow you to determine the improvement in strength of your pelvic floor muscles after consistent training (see page 76) for 3–6 weeks. Repeat the test once a week at the same time of day. Do not do it more often because the hormonal cycle and changes within your body may give false results. If after six weeks you have not improved in this test, go to a specialist women's health physiotherapist who is trained to guide you through the process of increasing the control over these muscles.

The blot challenge

1. Drink a glass of water and then empty your bladder. Two hours later, take a paper towel, fold in thirds, then in half, and place in your panties. With the paper towel in place, do 5 coughs; note the evidence of leakage from your bladder.

2. If you are dry, then do 5 astride jumps and recheck. So far so good?

3. Then repeat steps 1 and 2 together, i.e. cough and stride jump, and recheck.

(Many women will be wet by the second activity.)

This test (which is a fun coffee-group topic!) has been scientifically proven to be a reliable measure of stress incontinence and is reproducible, which means the size of the blot will clearly indicate the effectiveness of muscle training. If you become strong and quick in contracting your pelvic floor (exercise 3, page 76), practicing consistently, you may be surprised how effective this is.

TRAINING YOUR BLADDER

Do you know every toilet in town, and everyone close to you knows that you have to go FIRST to the toilet because you will always be busting? However funny to them, it is a most distressing situation to be in.

For a more long-term or complex problem with your bladder, you can evaluate your bladder habits by filling in a chart called a bladder diary (see page 127).

Using the bladder diary

Complete the chart over a week, recording with a simple check your fluid input (drinks), output (bathroom visits) and the time of each bathroom visit.

Record any leaks you may have (write "L" on the chart), or any urgent feelings ("U") that cause you distress (note that urgency is normal for some parts of our lives, when it is controllable).

Try to see the pattern of your fluid input / output. If you find you are having your drinks mostly in the early part of the day and going to the bathroom mostly in the afternoon, perhaps you could space this out more evenly through the day.

If you have leakage or urgency, look for what might be triggering these problems – sometimes bladder accidents are simply a result of drinking / bathroom habits developed over the years.

If your bladder is not under your control then try to train yourself to keep within the normal guidelines (see page 125). If you are uncertain about your diary results, check it out with a women's health physiotherapist.

BLADDER DIARY

Fluid:	SUN		MON		TUES		WED		THUR		FRI		SAT	
	Input	Output	Input	Output	Input	Output	Input	Output	Input	Output	Input	Output	Input	Output
6am														
7am														
8am														
9am														
10am														
11am														
12am														
1pm														
2pm														
3pm														
4pm														
5pm														
6pm														
7pm														
8pm														
9pm														
10pm														
11pm														
12pm														
1am														
2am														
3am														
4am														
5am														
TOTAL														

Unfortunately, there tends to be a genetic link to the risk of bladder prolapse. One theory is that the connective tissue, ligaments and smooth muscle that support us is more stretchy in some women. These also tend to get stretch marks, varicose veins and hemorrhoids.

If you know that you have a family history of bladder or uterus prolapse, talk to a women's health physiotherapist about how to manage that risk.

Some warnings for those at risk of prolapse:
*   Be careful about heavy lifting and straining.
*   Don't gain too much weight.
*   Don't get too tired and work too hard.
*   Don't strain to pass a bowel movement.
*   Don't cough uncontrollably (it places stress on your pelvic floor).
*   Be careful with exercises at the gym, always tighten your pelvic floor as you strain.
*   Don't have too many pregnancies carried to full term.
*   Keep as fit and healthy as possible, do not get run down.

Bladder repair surgery has a good success rate and for some women is very necessary to return them to a good quality of life. Your surgeon will tell you that there are some risks that you need to know about. Doing pelvic floor exercises (exercise 3, page 76) are ideal after a bladder repair operation and recommended by most specialists.

For a wide range of symptoms, two-thirds of women will be improved with pelvic floor exercises and bladder training. However, sometimes the bladder itself or the function of the muscle in its wall, called the detrusor, can be at fault. Conditions such as recurrent urinary tract infections, cystitis, vaginitis and

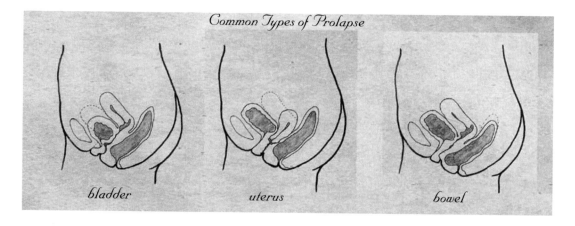

Common Types of Prolapse

bladder   uterus   bowel

endometriosis may be associated with urinary disturbances and pain in the mid-zone or lower torso. The medical treatment options of medication and non-invasive surgical procedures are well worth discussing with your doctor to restore your lifestyle to normal.

Bowel

If you are having problems with bowel leakage, you may need to concentrate on the bowel opening when doing pelvic floor exercises (exercise 3, page 76). Work on achieving a good squeeze or clamp action of this sphincter in isolation.

Difficulty with evacuating the bowel is often described by women as "fullness" of the bowel, which is not relieved with a normal bowel movement. Straining seems not to help as the bowel material remains "stuck," and often pressure with the fingers against the back wall of the vagina is the only relief. This is the classic description of a bowel prolapse or recto-cycele. If you feel you have similar symptoms, check with your doctor.

Hips and buttocks

A woman has wider hips and a narrower waist than a man and this pelvic shape causes an increase in all the angles and makes sweeping curves where the muscles have to work across the bones. If you place your hands at your side and slide them down to the outside of your thighs you come to some large bony points. These can become inflamed and the pain radiates from the muscles that attach in your buttock and run out to these bones.

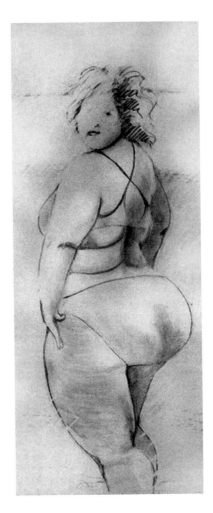

Hips may ache if you stand for periods of time; some women get sore hips if they walk a lot and pain in this region may be worse going up and down stairs. Sports where you bend over such as hockey, lunging in sports such as soccer and doing leg exercises at the gym, will subject the hips to stress which can cause pain and discomfort. Exercise 24, page 101, will help with this.

It actually requires a lot of work to lug our hips around or be sat upon all day. Your butt is a powerful muscle for driving your body forward and up and down stairs, lifting and general movement. Sitting on it all day doesn't offer much hope of keeping it in good shape – so what is the best butt, leg and pelvic exercise? Dancing of course.

Dancing is more than good exercise. There is social and spiritual energy given out in dance, which we need to put into our daily activities. Can you make the connection with your mind and body when you exercise? Perhaps there is an important aspect missing from your exercise, which, if added, will connect you to yourself. This means that you take pleasure in your exercise and the movement that you do through your day.

So why not put on music when you do housework, use the activity to get loose and burn some energy, take the walkman and play some great jazz when you walk or garden. If you really are too busy to go walking, try stepping on the spot.

When I was at home with my children when they were babies I always held them close and did lots of slow squats, and they loved it. It was my progressive resistance exercise – I would tighten my butt, pelvic floor and tummy as I came up from the squat and take big deep breaths. This helped to keep my lifting technique in good alignment, and as the babies got bigger and heavier, so I was getting stronger. It is also great for leg strengthening and for maintaining flexibility in the hip, knee and ankle joints.

Squatting

When you squat, go halfway only, knees bent to about 60–90 degrees.

Keep heels on the ground, let your body lean forward if you can and feel your hips and buttocks do the work. Breathe all the time, look straight ahead.

Maintain knee alignment over the second and third toe to avoid getting knee pain or kneecap irritation – don't be knock-kneed or bow-legged.

Build up to 20 squats 3 times a week.

Lunges, squats and walking would be my top three more regular lower limb exercises. They are not high impact, you can vary the speed, the number or time and you do not need weights.

Getting up from a chair

Don't use your arms and shoulders to push your body up from a chair – use your hips, legs and butt muscles and the momentum your body generates by leaning your nose over your toes. Keep your low back curve the same and drive up through your thighs. This is a great way not only to keep your muscles toned in your legs and butt, but to work on your balance. Try it five times for an extra workout. To make it easier, start with a higher chair such as a bar stool, and if your balance is a little wobbly for some reason, make sure you have a table in front of you for support.

There are many reasons for hip and buttock problems. Back pain and osteoarthritis are common causes of discomfort. If you suffer from these you should seek advice from a health professional to find out what is the best way for you to keep active.

Legs

People are an "upright, bipedal locomotor system," as my anatomy professor used to say. This means we are designed to move, walking around on two legs. We are happier when we are on the move because our body is at its most efficient. So what do we do? Sit at computers all day, drive around in cars and stand still for long periods.

Legs need to be walking; a little at a time and often enough so that the muscles in the legs are assisting the movement of fluid around your body. Thighs like to be worked to keep the knees strong for stair climbing, child lifting and vacuuming! And who doesn't want great legs that have nice shape and tone?

Think contractions, think pumping, think calf raises, and ankle movements.

Muscle contractions are needed to aid blood flow around the body and back to the heart. This type of muscle action resolves the problem associated with sitting still or in cramped positions and the possibility of clots forming in the veins of legs, for example during a long flight on an aircraft. Standing still for long periods can place your circulation at risk. Working on hard surfaces such as concrete can also play havoc with our legs and circulation.

Sluggish circulation can lead to a number of potential problems:

- cramp-like aches in legs and veins
- inflamed veins
- potential for blood clots

So if you sit still regularly, do the micromoves in sitting (see page 111).

Knees, ankles and feet

Many of us sag on our ankles and roll our feet either in or out (pronate or supinate), sometimes because of our shoes, sometimes due to weakness of our ankles. If you let the heels of shoes wear badly it allows the arches of the feet to get stretched, placing tension on the tendon at the back of the heel and making your feet ache. Perhaps we have had repeated ankle sprains or we may not have really thought about it. You can check what you do with your feet and ankles by looking at the wear pattern on the soles of your shoes or your footprints in the sand.

Correct stepping

When you step, the heel strike should be slightly on the outside of the heel; roll forward on your foot, then push off on the forefoot at the level of the second and third toes. It is not good for your feet if you push off through the big toe as it may cause bunions on the first joint.

Common problems with lower limbs are:

- *Achy and tired legs, especially if you are on your feet all day.*

- *Swollen ankles, from sitting still, legs crossed perhaps.*

- *Vein pressure – veins can actually hurt when they are inflamed and not working efficiently.*

Take care of your feet

Strengthen and tone the arches of your feet by drawing the arch of the foot up, holding for a few seconds, then relaxing.

Standing on one leg for 30 seconds strengthens the arch of the foot, the ankle, and helps balance.

Stand like a tripod on each foot – you need three key points of balance in both your feet to support your arch and align your body correctly all the way up. Keep the under surface or the pad of your big toe, the base or pad of your little toe and your heel on the floor. Now lift up your arch; try not to roll your ankles out as you do this. This is a static or isometric exercise, and is great for achy, tired legs.

Place your feet in good alignment and exercise the arches of your feet (as described above) whenever you are standing. Try to increase the amount of time you spend in this correct position.

Do the micromoves that specifically target feet and ankles (see page 111).

If you have persistent knee or ankle problems, or suspect a hip joint problem, there is more you need to know about, such as balance retraining, correct footwear and supports such as ankle braces or knee supports. An accurate diagnosis is advisable for persistent injury pain and weakness. While postural control helps with these joint problems, weight bearing such as simple walking may not be suitable. Exercise bike, aqua exercise or walking in water may be better for you, at least initially, while specific exercises need to be prescribed.

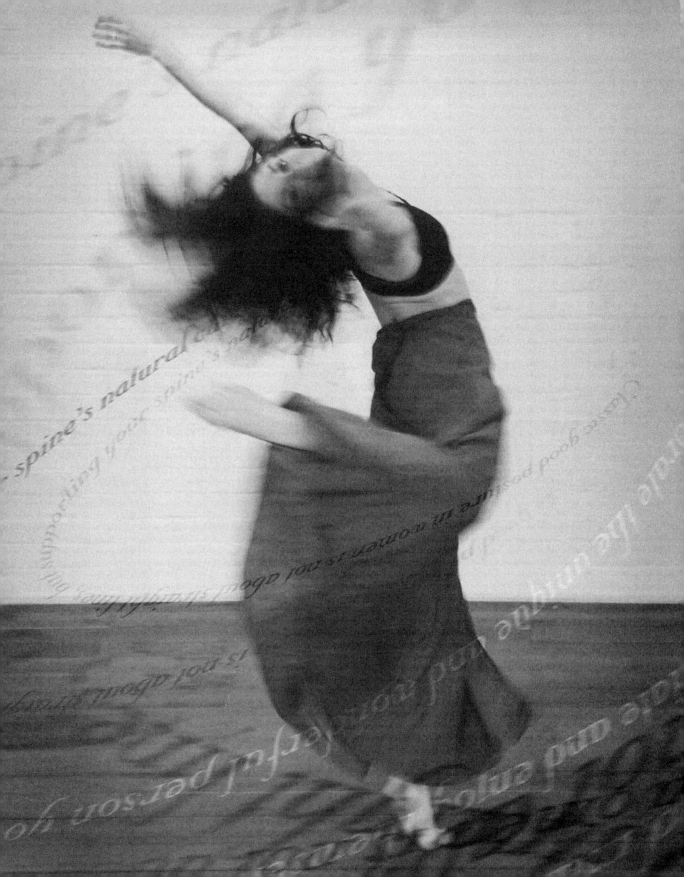

CONCLUSION

As a practicing physiotherapist, I am constantly reminded of issues that surround women today in relation to their bodies. Women often don't realize the impact of their posture on their body or how their wellbeing is tied to their body image. A manifestation of poor posture, such as back pain, headaches or limb pain can significantly affect how we feel, how we act and how we portray ourselves to the world, our partners and our children. Although many women know they have poor posture, how to alter it is something most feel is in the "too hard" basket. They believe they are too busy and that they would have to go to a gym or lose lots of weight or change themselves in some major way.

I saw the need for a book that my patients and friends could easily understand and use to help prevent and manage the problems that poor posture can bring, a book that said: "You can make the connection with your posture right now as you are reading, and start to celebrate the unique and wonderful person you are."

I wrote this book to encourage all women to appreciate and enjoy themselves and make simple beneficial changes that last for life. I knew that for me to make a difference, this book had to be easy to read, beautiful to look at, and touch the real woman of today – YOU.

Index

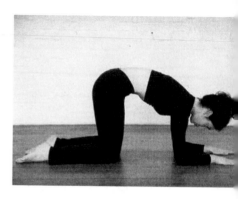

Exercises index

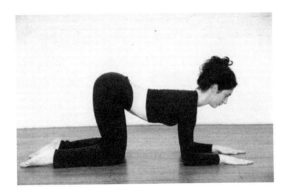

REFERENCES

Abrams, Paul, et al, "The Standardisation of Terminology of Lower Urinary Tract Function: Report from the Standardisation Sub-committee of the International Continence Society," *Neurology and Urodynamics,* 21: 167–178, 2002.

ACC and Core Services Committee statistics, 1996.

Interview with Ax, Maureen, Maureen Ax School of Dance, Palmerston North, New Zealand, 2002.

Hillary Commission, *Physical Activity Guidelines*, 1998.

Hooper, Anne, *The Kama Sutra,* Dorling Kindersley Publishers, London, 2000.

S. Kaplan, Helen, *New Sex Therapy,* Brunner-Routledge, New York, 1974.

Lacey, Hester, "Lessons in Sense and Sensuality, Belly dancing," *Independent on Sunday*, London, November 1995.

Interview with Pogson, Ian, MBChb, Diploma in Occupational Health, Director, Primary Corporate Health, 11 December 2002.

Regestein, Quentin R., "Sleep Disorders," *Clinical Psychiatry for Medical Students*, p 578; A. Stoudemire (editor). Lippincott, Philadelphia, 1990.

Rest, M.R.M. Tetley, in *Touch Physiotherapy Journal*, London, Summer 1997, no 84.

Roche Osteoporosis Advisory Panel. *Common Presentations of Osteoporosis.* In consultation with Dr Peter Dixon, Broadway Radiology, Palmerston North, New Zealand, 13 November 2002.

University of Washington Shoulder and Elbow Service – Patient Information – *5-1: Home Exercise Program for the Rough Shoulder.*

Other Books from Ulysses Press

ASHTANGA YOGA FOR WOMEN:
INVIGORATING MIND, BODY, AND SPIRIT WITH POWER YOGA
SALLY GRIFFYN, $17.95

Presents the exciting and empowering practice of power yoga in a balanced fashion that addresses the specific needs of female practitioners.

ELLIE HERMAN'S PILATES WORKBOOK ON THE BALL:
ILLUSTRATED STEP-BY-STEP GUIDE
ELLIE HERMAN, $13.95

Combines the powerful slimming and shaping effects of Pilates with the low-impact, high-intensity workout of the ball.

THE PILATES PRESCRIPTION FOR BACK PAIN: A COMPREHENSIVE PROGRAM
FOR DEVELOPING AND MAINTAINING A HEALTHY BACK
LYNNE ROBINSON, HELGE FISHER AND PAUL MASSEY, $14.95

While Pilates has recently become popular as a fitness trend, this book details the self-care program that applies the Pilates principles physical therapists have been using for decades to end back pain.

PILATES PERSONAL TRAINER BACK STRENGTHENING WORKOUT:
ILLUSTRATED STEP-BY-STEP MATWORK ROUTINE
MICHAEL KING AND YOLANDE GREEN, $9.95

The easy starter program in this workbook teaches Pilates exercises that are appropriate for strengthening the back in a safe and healthy manner.

PILATES PERSONAL TRAINER GETTING STARTED WITH STRETCHING:
ILLUSTRATED STEP-BY-STEP MATWORK ROUTINE
MICHAEL KING AND YOLANDE GREEN, $9.95

Ideal for beginners or older people, the specially designed Pilates exercises in this book offer a gentle workout of light strength movements and key stretches.

PILATES WORKBOOK:
ILLUSTRATED STEP-BY-STEP GUIDE TO MATWORK TECHNIQUES
MICHAEL KING, $12.95

Illustrates the core matwork movements exactly as Joseph Pilates intended them to be performed; readers learn each movement by following the photographic sequences and explanatory captions.

PILATES WORKBOOK FOR PREGNANCY:
ILLUSTRATED STEP-BY-STEP MATWORK TECHNIQUES
MICHAEL KING AND YOLANDE GREEN, $12.95

Presented in an easy-to-use style with step-by-step photo sequences of Pilates matwork techniques – adapted here for pregnancy and post-pregnancy.

WEIGHT-BEARING WORKOUTS FOR WOMEN:
EXERCISES FOR SCULPTING, STRENGTHENING & TONING
YOLANDE GREEN, $12.95

Weight training is the fastest, most effective way to lose fat, improve muscle tone and strengthen bones. This workbook shows just how easy it is for women at any age to get started with weights.

WEIGHTS ON THE BALL WORKBOOK:
STEP-BY-STEP GUIDE WITH OVER 350 PHOTOS
STEVEN STIEFEL, $14.95

With exercises suited for all skill levels, *Weights on the Ball Workbook* shows how to simultaneously use weights and the exercise ball for the ultimate total-body workout.

YOGA IN FOCUS: POSTURES, SEQUENCES, AND MEDITATIONS
JESSIE CHAPMAN   PHOTOGRAPHS BY DHYAN, $14.95

A beautiful celebration of yoga that's both useful for learning the techniques and inspiring in its artistic approach to presenting the body in yoga positions.

YOGA FOR PARTNERS: OVER 75 POSTURES TO DO TOGETHER
JESSIE CHAPMAN   PHOTOGRAPHS BY DHYAN, $14.95

An excellent tool for learning two-person yoga, *Yoga for Partners* features inspiring photos of the paired asanas. It teaches each partner how to synchronize their movements and breathing, bringing new lightness and enjoyment to any yoga practice.

YOGA FOR 50+: MODIFIED POSES & TECHNIQUES FOR A SAFE PRACTICE
RICHARD ROSEN, $14.95

As baby boomers pass age 50, problems with knees, ankles and backs are leading them into lower-impact forms of fitness. Tailored specifically for this burgeoning population, *Yoga for 50+* offers a straightforward approach that makes it easy to learn yoga at any age.

To order these books call 800-377-2542 or 510-601-8301, fax 510-601-8307, e-mail ulysses@ulyssespress.com, or write to Ulysses Press, P.O. Box 3440, Berkeley, CA 94703. All retail orders are shipped free of charge. California residents must include sales tax. Allow two to three weeks for delivery.

Carol Armitage specializes in women's health, running a physiotherapy clinic and conducting public workshops. She also has extensive clinical experience working with international athletes. **Mike Bebb** lectures at Massey University and runs the Centre for Vision and Leadership. Both live in New Zealand.

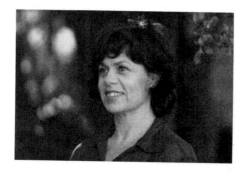

Carol Armitage